MORE PRAISE FOR
Social Networks and Popular Understanding of Science and Health: Sharing Disparities

"Southwell is a leading expert on communication about science and health. This book is necessary reading for anyone interested in human survival and well-being and how communication through mass media and via social networks affects both."

— James Druckman, Professor of Political Science at Northwestern University and former editor of Public Opinion Quarterly

"An absorbing book. Southwell eloquently explains what few will have realized: that the explosion of opportunities to share knowledge through social media appears to exacerbate disparities in public understanding of health and science, rather than level the field. He challenges us to think more deeply about strategies for public communication that would prevent those most socioeconomically disadvantaged from being left even further behind."

— Melanie Wakefield, Director, Centre for Behavioural Research in Cancer, Cancer Council Victoria, Melbourne, Australia

"Southwell provides critical frameworks and findings regarding health and social media. Digitally enabled by social media tools, peer-to-peer connections can help amplify voices by shaping health content and user experiences."

— Fay Cobb Payton, Associate Professor of Information Systems, North Carolina State University, and Founder and Director of My Health Impact Network

Social Networks and Popular Understanding of Science and Health: Sharing Disparities

Brian G. Southwell

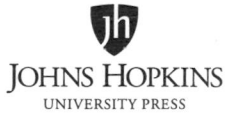

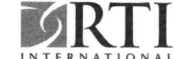

Library of Congress Control Number: 2013944860

ISBN 978-1-4214-1324-2 (pbk.: alk. paper)
ISBN 978-1-4214-1325-9 (electronic)
ISBN 1-4214-1324-8 (pbk.: alk. paper)
ISBN 1-4214-1325-6 (electronic)

RTI Press publication No. BK-0011-1307
doi:10.3768/rtipress.2013.bk.0011.1307

RTI International is an independent, nonprofit research organization dedicated to improving the human condition by turning knowledge into practice. RTI offers innovative research and technical services to governments and businesses worldwide in the areas of health and pharmaceuticals, education and training, surveys and statistics, advanced technology, international development, economic and social policy, energy and the environment, and laboratory testing and chemistry services.

The Johns Hopkins University Press
2715 North Charles Street, Baltimore, MD 21218-4363 USA
www.press.jhu.edu

This publication is part of the RTI Press Book series.
RTI International
3040 East Cornwallis Road, PO Box 12194, Research Triangle Park, NC 27709-2194 USA
rtipress@rti.org
www.rti.org

Dedication

To my own social network, especially Jessica, Gavin, and my family, for all that they share with me.

Contents

Acknowledgments   vii

Chapter 1. Introduction   1

    Discussion Goals   3

    How This Book Is Structured   4

    Acknowledging Disparities in Information Sharing 5

Chapter 2. Evidence of Inequality in Information Sharing   7

    Conversation Gaps   8

    Interpersonal Interaction: Everyday Occurrence and a Marketing Tool   10

    Social Science Observation of Information Diffusion: A Tendency Toward Disparities   12

    Differences Versus Disparities   13

    Summary   15

Chapter 3. A Catalogue of Information-Sharing Behaviors   17

    Social Networks and Relevant Principles   17

    Conversation (or Talk)   22

    Forwarding   24

    Overt Endorsement   25

    Commentary and Cooptation   26

    Referral   27

    Theoretical Comparison of Information-Sharing Behaviors   27

    Summary   29

Chapter 4. Who One Is Matters: Individual-Level Factors
That Affect Sharing   31

    Socioeconomic Status   33

    Education   34

    Perceived Topical Relevance   36

    Perceived Understanding   37

    Personality   39

    Communication Apprehension and Shyness   40

    Sensation Seeking   41

    The Limits of Individual Differences   44

Chapter 5. Where One Is Matters: Community-Level Factors
That Affect Sharing   47

    The Effects of Network Characteristics   49

Social Capital, Social Cohesion, and Available Community Ties 51

Why Community Ties Should Affect Information Sharing 54

Community Endurance and Residential Stability 56

Community Ties, Stability, and Peer Referral for Mammography: An Empirical Example 56

Relationship History 57

Cultural Differences 59

The Need for Contextual Understanding 62

Chapter 6. What Information Matters: Content-Level Factors That Affect Sharing 63

Does Rhetorical Structure Matter? 68

Is There a Role for Emotional Response? 70

Can Messages Boost Confidence in Talking With Others? 72

Incentive Offers for Peer Referral 74

The Case for Message-Level Differences 75

Chapter 7. The Consequences of Information Sharing 77

Knowledge Gain 79

Cognitive Salience 81

Social Norm Awareness 85

Conferral of Argument Resistance 88

The Consequences of Social Network Interaction 89

Chapter 8. Remedies and Realism 93

Why Are Information-Sharing Disparities Problematic? 93

How Can Disparities Be Remedied? 96

Boost Collective Confidence 97

Meet People Where They Are 98

Build Community Connection Infrastructure 99

Acknowledging Disparities While Moving Forward 103

References 107

About the Author 131

Index 133

Acknowledgments

This book reflects a sense of urgency that I developed over several years as it became apparent that our networked future won't guarantee the equity that some suggest it will. The task of bringing that vague sense of urgency to a point of sufficient coherence to be shared required collective effort, and I am grateful for the help I received. A number of collaborators and students have produced study results that I summarize in the book and I share credit for those ideas with them. Many of the central insights I have had about the role of social networks in mass communication flow stem from lunches with my dear friend Marco Yzer. Some of these thoughts, in fact, can be traced back to my own doctoral work with the incomparable Bob Hornik and the exceptional faculty at the University of Pennsylvania.

After landing in North Carolina in 2011, I had the good fortune to connect with the RTI Press team. Karen Lauterbach, Diane Wagener, and Dorota Temple were all early champions of the idea of the book and I am grateful for that; Karen also has been a patient and helpful Managing Editor. Associate Editor Ina Wallace and a set of anonymous peer reviewers helped shape the book into its current form, and I appreciate their efforts. Jeffrey Novey, Joanne Studders, Anne Gering, Tayo Jolaoso, Kit Wienert, Alisa Clifford, Rodica Simon, and Chad Stinner, among others, provided exceptional copyediting, graphics, and layout support.

I also am grateful to have found a place like RTI International, where people like Lauren McCormack, Amy Roussel, and Janet Mitchell actively encourage public engagement through scholarship. Kelley Squazzo of Johns Hopkins University Press has been an enthusiastic and insightful advocate for the book, and Martha Sewall helped develop the final version of the cover. Colleagues at the University of North Carolina at Chapel Hill and Duke University also have provided helpful feedback on earlier versions of these ideas, as have colleagues around the country and globe. Beyond professional assistance, my family provided support, understanding, and even ideas beyond what anyone reasonably could request as I spent late nights, car trips, and time at the beach thinking about and finishing the book. They inspire me.

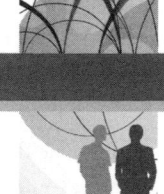

CHAPTER 1

Introduction

In June 2012, the United States Supreme Court announced a milestone decision regarding health policy, upholding major tenets of the Patient Protection and Affordable Care Act (Affordable Care Act). The Act ensures increased access to health coverage for many Americans and introduces new protections for people with health insurance. Ironically, the ways that news about the Court's decision spread among people underscores the information inequality facing the nation. As this landmark decision was announced, many citizens learned about the news directly from television or radio reports or over the Internet. Despite prominent broadcast by media outlets, many other people first learned about the news from coworkers they passed in the hall or colleagues at a meeting who had happened to hear the news. Yet other people tried to make sense of the complex legal decision by talking with friends or family members. Some Americans, however, did not hear the details of the Court's decision at all that morning, and neither did anyone they happened to see that day.

Within hours of the Court's decision, some people were actively debating the nuances of the health care policy itself or forecasting the impact of the decision's framing on the 2012 presidential election. Others were able to solicit expert advice as to whether the decision had any direct impact on their use of health care services or on their pocketbook. Other people did not enjoy the benefit of chatting with neighbors or friends about what the decision meant. For some people, this lack of conversational focus on health policy was an active choice. Given the opportunity to talk about any topic during a work break, last night's sports scores or the latest celebrity scandal likely seemed much more appealing than the subtleties of an individual mandate to purchase health insurance.

For some people, however, forces had been set in motion prior to that morning that ensured that the social network in which they reside would not actively interact to share, discuss, or forward news about the Court's decision. Chances are that those people went to sleep the night following the historic decision with little more than a vague awareness that something in Washington, DC, had happened that day involving President Obama and health insurance. The social amplification of understanding and opinion that quickly unfolded that day for some people left others relatively in the dark and undisturbed.

Polling conducted soon after the health care decision revealed the extent to which prevalent broadcast of health and science news does not necessarily result in widespread understanding. Within weeks of the Court's ruling, a striking gap in public understanding came to light. Nearly half of survey respondents were confused as to the basic facts of the decision. About one-third of respondents were unaware of the details of the case and about another 15 percent actually reported that the Affordable Care Act was overturned by the Supreme Court.[1] Many different factors likely produced that unevenness in understanding. One set of possible factors, nonetheless, involves the people with whom respondents interact (or do not interact) regularly. While *social network interaction* certainly cannot account for all aspects of this uneven state of knowledge, a dearth of health policy knowledge within a person's immediate network may contribute to this gap or to the echo chamber effect that polarized, ideologically charged network discussion may have had on erroneous interpretation of news coverage. Consequently, the importance of social networks is a main focus of this book.

The example of information sharing regarding the Affordable Care Act begins to show how the effect of social network interaction on information spread is not solely dictated by the sheer volume of information broadcast from a central source. In other words, social network interaction is not merely uniform rippling following a stone cast in the information pond. It appears that some ponds are more receptive than others; that is, some networks are primed to engage broadcast news, whereas others are not.

Consider a news example contemporary to the Affordable Care Act that may be, scientifically speaking, even more fundamental and profound as an advance in human knowledge: the announcement in summer 2012 of evidence consistent with the existence of the Higgs boson, what many journalists dubbed the "God particle."[2] The discovery generated substantial news coverage in Europe and around the world. Subsequently, some social networks simmered with not only general references to the news but also jokes and puns and commentary. An example that bounced around Facebook involved a Higgs boson disrupting a Catholic church service exclaiming, "Wait! You can't have mass without me!" The sum effect of such simmering likely kept the news salient for many people. However, without a basic background in physics or access to colleagues who had one, other people apparently did not witness much social interaction regarding the topic at all.

Discussion Goals

One goal of this book is to document gaps between groups of people in their tendency to share information about health and science. Documenting such disparities is important to correct popular misperceptions regarding the free and unfettered flow of information that supposedly abounds in the present moment. Pundits and scholars talk about the emergence of the information age in the 21st century.[3] Central to such conceptualizations is the grand promise of peer-to-peer sharing. That is, instead of living in a *one-to-many* broadcast era, we live in an environment in which information can be expressed from *many to many* 24 hours a day. But the inference that all are sharing equally in this feast does not entirely jibe with empirical reality. While some celebrate the potential of social media and other new peer-to-peer connection technologies for teaching people about science and health in this century, enthusiasm about peer-to-peer information flow requires important caveats. Rather than encouraging equity in what we all know and think about scientific discoveries, household consumer tips, the latest health recommendations or opportunities for medical services, systematic reliance on social networks to spread information may be a recipe for inequity.

As delineated in these pages, an increasing body of research suggests that people are not equal in their tendency to share information with others around them. In general, people do not take advantage of the chance to share ideas with others, a paradox in our current era of apparent information abundance. But it also appears that some people are much less likely than others to share information. Some of the differences in peer-to-peer sharing represent inequity in that information sharing is constrained unjustly by factors outside of a person's immediate control. This book explains why these information-sharing patterns appear to persist, why it matters to society, and what, if anything, can be done to address these tendencies.

This exploration is relevant to everyday citizens as well as to those involved in public policy debates about the appropriate tools for large-scale educational efforts in a variety of topical domains. The book also will appeal to social science students interested in the role of social networks in explaining information diffusion. Additionally, this is a cautionary tale for communication practitioners, such as informal education specialists or health promotion professionals, interested in leveraging social ties as an inexpensive method to spread information.

Our discussion will focus specifically on information about human health and other large-scale scientific research funded and conducted at an institutional level, given that popular understanding of those areas of knowledge can impact both individual well-being and collective decision-making about public policy. At the same time, we can learn a great deal from social science research on information diffusion and engagement related to other (not entirely distinct) topics, such as politics and popular culture, and consequently also will draw in that evidence where appropriate. Focusing the discussion in this way does not imply that health and science are unique in being vulnerable to information-sharing disparities, though the preponderance of highly specialized knowledge in these domains and Americans' performance on knowledge assessments[4-6] do suggest that these topics are especially relevant for consideration of social networks and information flow.

How This Book Is Structured

The structure of the book is fourfold. In Chapters 2 and 3, I discuss evidence that gaps in information sharing exist and describe different types of information-sharing activities (such as face-to-face conversation and electronic message forwarding) in which such disparities should be evident theoretically. Then it will be important to extensively consider *why* information-sharing differences occur and to address the potential need for remedies.

In Chapters 4 through 6, I describe a series of relevant studies and explanations for information-sharing and information-spread disparities. Almost any difference between individual people could be noteworthy from a communication strategy perspective. However, as we will see, some of the reasons people may be unequal in their propensity to share information with others will be both logical and yet, to some observers, unremarkable from an ethical perspective. As I will discuss, the fact that some people harbor personality traits that make them less outgoing may not be cause for concern about their reduced tendency to pass along news that they see on television to other people. Other factors, though, will suggest discrepancy between the well-being or preferences of people and what happens in reality that reflects potentially avoidable structural barriers to sharing or receiving truthful and useful information from peers. For example, people in a neighborhood may all benefit from information about environmental harm being caused by a local factory, but the lack of established connections between neighbors may reduce the spread of news that one person in that neighborhood happens to receive about that harm. That latter pattern, relative to information sharing that we might witness in a more socially connected neighborhood, may trigger a sense of injustice or at least cause for concern.

In Chapter 7, I engage the question of why we should worry about such disparities from an ethical perspective and at the same time acknowledge the critique that some types of inequalities likely matter more than others. Admittedly, the discussion will not consistently highlight reasons for information-sharing differences that warrant alarm. Not all of the discussion will focus on inequity; some of what we will witness simply holds practical implication for outreach that relies on peer-to-peer information campaigns. Nonetheless, some readers also will find other examples that do signal need for intervention.

Finally, in Chapter 8, I describe what, if anything, can be done to address these patterns of information sharing.

Acknowledging Disparities in Information Sharing

By considering a range of our daily interactions with other people, we can start to understand how it is that two people may have roughly an equal chance to see a particular story on the morning television news and yet, over the course of a day, may end up with very different knowledge, beliefs, and behaviors relative to the topic of that story because of the influence of others around them. It is important to note that, as I will discuss in Chapter 2, anyone with access to the Internet now has access to a wealth of information relative to people living in earlier centuries. Technical access, however, is not equivalent to routine engagement. Here the discussion will focus on social interactions and the way that interpersonal information sources supplement (or do not supplement) the stream of information people choose (or are able) to engage on their own in listening to or viewing mass media outlets or subscribing to information services in isolation from other people.

By focusing on information sharing between people, we will see why some types of information are simply more likely to be shared than others, regardless of individual differences between people. We also will explore how it is that some people simply never get exposed at all to otherwise seemingly prominent information. Research has started to point to a number of reasons why people have different routine interpersonal experiences when it comes to information about health, science, and myriad other topics. We can take stock of that research and related theory and see that it forecasts a society in which the mere broadcasting of a message is not sufficient to guarantee information equity across all people.

People have sought and obtained information from a variety of sources for thousands of years; before television there was the town crier, and people have been talking to one another as long as there has been human speech. Throughout hundreds of years of mass communication history, some people have been more connected to the latest developments in human health and scientific research than others, at least partially because of well-informed people that they know who share information with those in their social circle. What is striking about the present moment, however, is that many people believe communication technology offers great democratic promise that can help overcome some of the disparities that have divided us. But as we will discuss, we are far from enjoying universal access to new communication technologies[7,8] and even increased access to those technologies will not automatically overcome the network tendencies of human groups in which some tend to be more connected than others. A central paradox ultimately will animate this discussion: the notion that while we live in a world that is awash in information and increasingly filled with exuberant references to "social networks," the very network infrastructure that stems from our social nature can lead to the reification and amplification of disparities between people with each new release of information into the system.

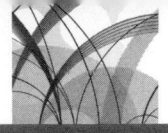
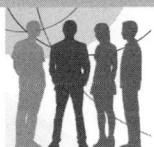

CHAPTER 2

Evidence of Inequality in Information Sharing

The catastrophe in New Orleans and the surrounding region associated with Hurricane Katrina in 2005 lays bare some of the differences in information access that stem simply from who one knows. The natural disaster, compounded by failures in the city's built infrastructure, garnered major news coverage for weeks. A story that did not receive as much attention involved the peer-to-peer information sharing, or lack thereof, that happened among city residents. One study, for example, analyzed survey data gathered from more than 400 respondents in Houston, Texas, shelters a couple of weeks after the storm hit the coast.[1] These respondents had been living in New Orleans and were moved to the Houston shelters in the days and weeks after the hurricane made landfall. The study found that respondents who reported not having local networks of family and friends in New Orleans on whom they could depend were less likely to even have received official information about the evacuation warning than were others. In other words, those without dependable social networks reported less access to potentially life-altering information.

Another example highlights the way in which one's social network matters as a predictor of one's everyday information diet: social network interaction often helps to amplify differences between people in the valence or *framing* of information that people read or hear. In 2009, the United States was in the midst of the H1N1 influenza virus pandemic. During the latter months of that year, scientists developed a promising vaccine for mass distribution. What transpired on social media, however, is a story that went underreported by news outlets at the time and is especially telling. As Salathé and Khandelwal[2] elegantly demonstrated, publicly available Twitter feeds revealed a divided nation. This study looked at feeds from more than 100,000 Twitter users to attempt to understand whether sentiments regarding the new vaccine suggested clustering such that people of particular viewpoints tended to be connected. (Imagine a feather as an opinion, and the old adage about birds of a feather flocking together artfully describes the clustering phenomenon.) The findings showed that regions of the country where correspondent Twitter messages tended to mention the H1N1 vaccine in a *positive* context also tended to have higher flu vaccination rates according to separate US Centers for Disease Control and Prevention data. Regions where sentiment was relatively more *negative* tended also to have lower flu vaccination rates.

Twitter posts are not novels. They are limited to 140 characters or less, so they are pithy at best and abbreviated and difficult to comprehend at worst. Nonetheless, Salathé and Khandelwal were able to code posts as being at least positive, negative, or neutral. The results suggest that not only does interaction via social media reflect correspondent behavior offline but also that noteworthy differences exist in people's behavior that are detectable as a function of online social networks. Moreover, the results revealed a distinctly polarized nation with little information flow *between* well-vaccinated groups and less-vaccinated groups. Not only were most communities measured in the study essentially dominated by positive or negative sentiment (rather than organized around neutral sentiment), but, based on analysis of those following and responding to various Twitter posts, it also appears that people who felt negatively about the vaccine were unlikely to engage in any discernible way with people who felt positively about the vaccine and vice versa.

Conversation Gaps

The example of Hurricane Katrina suggests that we live in a society characterized by distinct gaps in knowledge between what may be labeled the information haves and the information have-nots. Such a sociological phenomenon is not new, as it was documented decades ago in the United States with work to explore the so-called knowledge gap hypothesis.[3] The Katrina and H1N1 examples also suggest that we may live in a society characterized by real and consequential *conversation gaps*. Simply stated, some corners of society should be predictably more likely to talk about announcements, campaigns, and other news items. Not only should the simple presence or absence of conversation vary, but we also are likely to see sentiment polarization such that the dominant norms of discussion on various topics contrast sharply.

The original work on the knowledge gap hypothesis[3] found support for a relatively simple and logical, but nonetheless important, hypothesis: people who already hold knowledge about a particular topic will be more likely to glean new topical information over time from mass media. In other words, people rich in information are likely to get richer for various reasons related to information processing. More recently, Viswanath and Finnegan[4] forecasted that existing gaps between the information rich and poor will continue to be exacerbated, not ameliorated, by mass media exposure over time because access to, and the technical nature of, much current information will benefit the information rich disproportionately. Such gaps are particularly problematic in arenas, such as health and science, in which equal holding of knowledge otherwise could help to equalize overall well-being.[5]

The knowledge gap literature and more recent work on interpersonal communication converge to suggest a specific disparity in talk about health and science. We should expect exposure to mass media content not to simply produce learning, persuasion, or reinforcement. Societal exposure to mass media should stimulate relevant conversation among social networks. Importantly, the basic potential for conversation or other forms of information sharing likely is not uniform for all audiences. The potential for sharing will vary between people in terms of tendency, amount, and content. That variance, in turn, widens gaps between people over time. In a world in which peer-to-peer information sharing is facilitated by technology and encouraged by campaign professionals, we can forecast an information environment characterized by disparity, polarization, and discrepancy.

Apparent disparity and disjuncture is paradoxical given the popular description of the world as a highly interconnected place, particularly with regard to electronic media. We live in a world infiltrated and connected by electronic media. Some have argued that most people in societies similar to the United States now swim in a daily "torrent" of information unlike any witnessed on Earth before.[6] Gleick[7] has taken the weather metaphor further, describing our information age as nothing short of a "flood." Much of that information is potentially beneficial. In the 21st century United States and elsewhere around the world, we live in moments characterized by a tremendous amount of practical and useful information about how a person can improve their individual health, about how a family can improve its well-being, and about how communities can forge ahead in sustainable ways. Nonetheless, our tendencies to cohabitate, collaborate, and conspire with other people—in other words, our highly social nature as humans—complicate the extent to which we can live in a society united solely by broadcast mass media messages.

On some level, this is a healthy aspect of societal infrastructure; being connected to one another interpersonally helps to ensure that we are not subject to the authoritarian whims of a central set of elites. The very strength of the Internet lies in its replication of our tendency toward decentralized webs of social networks rather than a society built around a single hub. However, the role of social networks in the dissemination and effects of broadcast information is multidimensional. There is a downside to this network infrastructure. In short, networks vary, for myriad reasons, including their willingness, ability, and tendency to interact regarding information about health and science. That variance is theoretically predictable and yet it also has important consequences for anyone concerned with the state of science knowledge or what people believe about various health topics in the United States.

Interpersonal Interaction: Everyday Occurrence and a Marketing Tool

We interact with one another in many ways, and of course have done so long before Charles Babbage's calculating machine ushered in the contemporary computing era. In fact, we typically interact so frequently that it is easy to overlook the sheer prevalence of the behavior in our everyday lives. Research suggests that most people directly interact with other people in some fashion more often than they engage virtually any mass media outlet; for example, people talk to other people far more often than they read newspapers or watch television.[8,9] Each interaction holds the potential to share vital information. Talking with other people may teach you about how best to protect yourself in the event of a flu outbreak. Someone forwarding a magazine article on energy-saving tips for your home may provide a wealth of information. A disapproving look from a loved one may discourage you from drinking more alcohol than you have already consumed one evening. You may even learn the latest information about a natural disaster unfolding in your town.[10]

Within professional advertising and marketing circles, reliance on interpersonal networks as tools for diffusion has been au courant for a number of years. One need not look further than the proliferation in the past two decades of buzz words and concepts, such as viral marketing, word-of-mouth advertising, or viral communication.[11-15] These terms refer to the practice of getting consumers to tell other people about products or ideas; an example would be handing out stacks of coupons for free tickets to a science museum to current customers in the hopes that they would share them with friends or family. Montgomery[12] described viral marketing as "a type of marketing that infects its customers with an advertising message, which passes from one customer to the next like a rampant flu virus" (p. 93). The enthusiasm of Phelps and colleagues[13] was familiar to many commercial advertisers when they emphasized the possibilities of engaging consumer networks directly and encouraging people to pass along information to others they know as an alternative to solely using mass media strategies. Viral marketing efforts attempt to mobilize existing social networks.[16] Such efforts can involve outcomes as diverse as commercial sales and political campaigns, but at their core most viral marketing efforts depend on individuals sharing information with (and about) family and friends. The success of a viral marketing approach depends on the willingness and ability of individuals to share goods, services, and ideas with others in their network.

In recent years, enthusiasm for the potential of viral marketing is on the rise among not only commercial advertisers or politicians but also nonprofit professionals and social marketing professionals. For example, after assessing efforts to promote health in Tanzania using radio soap operas, Mohammed[17] advocated for public health officials to engage social networks as a way to "turbocharge" their campaign efforts. On a similar note, Gladwell[18] wrote of "word-of-mouth epidemics" as he attempted to explain the flow of information among populations.* As a matter of routine practice, strategists now actively recruit people who appear to be key information hubs to endorse certain messages and to pass along information to others in their social networks. In one example of a randomized controlled trial among health care providers, Lomas and colleagues[19] found that intervening to encourage physicians to share information with colleagues about the value of vaginal births among women who had previously had a Cesarean-section delivery dramatically increased adoption of the practice. The study documented an increase of approximately 85 percent in vaginal birth delivery among post-Cesarean women over time. In another example, L'Engle and colleagues[20] reported that approximately a fifth of program participants for a reproductive health project conducted in Tanzania found out about the project through friends or family who had been in contact in some fashion with the program originally. Consequently, working with people to spread messages to people they know is a popular strategy for many professionals from Madison Avenue to Minneapolis and around the world. But to what end might this approach lead?

---

* The recursive coincidence of *viral* metaphors with actual public health efforts to improve infectious disease preparedness through word-of-mouth techniques is not likely random.

Social Science Observation of Information Diffusion: A Tendency Toward Disparities

At least since the French sociologist Gabriel Tarde's observation[21] in 1903 of our human tendency to imitate others and thus to transmit behaviors and ideas, researchers have been intrigued by the widespread propagation of ideas through society. Many accounts of that propagation have involved peer-to-peer transmission in some form. The appearance of Katz and Lazarsfeld's *Personal Influence*[22] in 1955 helped to popularize the idea that ideas may pass from mass media outlets through popular opinion leaders and on to those who are linked socially to those opinion leaders. In a sense, people are a vector for idea transmission.

Later thinking about the popularization of beliefs conceptualized an idea itself as a unit with some degree of agency, or at least momentum and trajectory, relative to people who serve as a medium. In 1976, in *The Selfish Gene*, Dawkins[23] coined the notion of a meme, a conceptual analog of a gene, replete with the potential for extinction or replication and dependent on person-to-person transmission (along with broadcast via mass media) for survival over time. A meme is a short and pithy expression of an idea, such as the question "Where's the beef?" in the 1980s* or references to "Gangnam style" starting in 2012.†

The long line of academic thinking about information diffusion via interpersonal interaction is relevant insofar as it suggests that some types and presentations of information show more promise than others for replication and diffusion. We even may be able to craft recommendations for overcoming disparities in diffusion by paying attention to theorizing about memes. Nonetheless, precious few memes enjoy universal residence among everyone, and so the story we will explore in this book will be, at least in part, about the myriad complications that appear to favor science and health idea propagation in some networks rather than others. Studying information propagation potential leads to the literature on interpersonal interactions between people. It also affords a view of differences between communities in the amount and type of such interactions as well as differences between messages in their ability to travel through society.

---

* The phrase began as a catchphrase in a 1984 Wendy's fast food restaurant television commercial and later was used by presidential candidate Walter Mondale in a debate.

† The neologism describes upscale fashion and lifestyle associated with a section of Seoul, South Korea, and was popularized by the musical artist PSY.

Part of the justification for the arguments presented in this book lies in observations of the wider world outside of social science laboratories set up to investigate interactions between people. The prospect of social networks tending toward disproportionate concentration of information-sharing activity among a few rather than uniformly across an entire population actually is what we would expect based on the literature on networks in myriad facets of the natural world.[24-27] Newman's work[25,28] on a phenomenon known as preferential attachment is especially revealing in this regard. Newman[28] pointed out that evidence of preferential attachment is everywhere, from the growth and distribution of blood vessels in the body to hyperlinks in the World Wide Web. Essentially, new linkages are most likely to form as attachments to already well-connected hubs. Over time, the most well-connected hubs will attract even more connections than less well-connected hubs.

In other words, consistent observation of preferential attachment suggests that purely egalitarian connection networks are not the rule; instead, we tend to see clustering. This partly reflects the development of networks that arise as attachments grow in response to an already existing resource. When a child arrives on the playground, for instance, she will notice that there are some clusters of children already playing together at the jungle gym or on the soccer field; typically, children are not uniformly distributed equidistantly from one another. I have observed a similar phenomenon unfold at an outdoor concert at which there were rather long lines for the portable bathroom facilities closest to the concert venue that grew as people blindly queued where others had lined up, whereas only a few feet away a line of facilities stood virtually empty and remained so largely because people had somehow assumed they needed to gather where other people had first started gathering. Similarly, as a person becomes known as a purveyor of information, she or he will be an attractive force when a new person, or node, enters the system. People notice active sources and tend to gather where others have gathered already.

Differences Versus Disparities

Reasonable people can debate the ethical implications of the landscape in this book, which is not uniform in the flow of information between people but rather marked with distinct obstacles and constraints. While our tendency toward this landscape is empirically evident in myriad ways we will discuss in these pages, whether the pattern warrants any worry or intervention is a question that will invite some discord between observers. We can inform such a debate, at least, by acknowledging at the outset that a conceptual distinction can be drawn between differences and disparities.

To draw such a distinction, we can take a cue from research and commentary on disparities in population health. Margaret Whitehead,[29] a consultant for the World Health Organization writing in a widely cited paper on inequity in health, has noted that "there is bound to be some natural variation between one individual and another"; and goes on to state that "[w]e will never be able to achieve a situation where everyone in the population has the same level of health … and dies after exactly the same life span" (p. 219). From Whitehead's perspective, and consistent with a long line of disparity scholars following her,[30,31] we can draw distinctions between the simple fact of difference and considerations of factors that produce differences that are potentially avoidable, unnecessary, or somehow unjust.

More recently, Paula Braveman's efforts to define health disparities as a concept provided additional insight on information-sharing disparities. Specifically, Braveman[32] asserted that health disparities are "potentially avoidable differences in health … between groups of people who are more and less advantaged socially" (p. 180). In other words, Braveman emphasized both the importance of avoidable differences and social disadvantage in defining differences that matter sufficiently to count as disparities.

Some examples may help to illustrate what can be counted as disparity with regard to health. Vivier and colleagues[33] used data from the Rhode Island Department of Health to demonstrate that where a child resides plays a major role in determining their likelihood of experiencing lead poisoning. They found that children living in the poorest neighborhoods and in the oldest housing were more likely than others to have elevated blood lead levels. Given the role of lead in dampening children's development, this pattern is one that seems to perpetuate differences in a manner that is beyond a child's own choices or control. Watson and colleagues[34] found that relatively poor North Carolina residents tended to live in areas that objectively perform relatively poorly on environmental health indicators. At the same time, they found a disconnect between residents' perceived and objective risk, such that perceived risks were predicted by local television news viewing more than by objective risk measures for their area of residence. The fact that poorer residents were somewhat blind to the environmental risks in their own backyard struck the authors as an instance of injustice. Similarly, in conceptualizing disparities in science and health-information sharing, perhaps we ought to be most concerned about instances of information-sharing differences that appear to be driven by social standing or to result in discrepancy in knowledge or understanding among socially disadvantaged groups relative to more advantaged members of society.

Summary

This brief tour through research on information flow yields at least three salient observations. First, we can find numerous instances in which people vary dramatically in their engagement with information about science and health as a function of their social networks. Second, information, like elements of many other networks, does not propagate and spread uniformly; some people tend to be distribution hubs more than others and some pieces of information are more likely to travel than others—an idea expanded on in Chapter 3 where we look more directly at the notion of a "social network." Third, some types of information-sharing differences are more problematic than others, an idea examined in Chapter 7. Having described this uneven landscape, the next logical question is how these disparities come to be. Chapters 4, 5, and 6 explore a variety of factors that predict differences in information sharing between people.

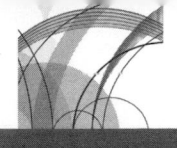

CHAPTER 3

A Catalogue of Information-Sharing Behaviors

When considering how information about health and science spreads, resonates, and spurs behavior, interactions between people appear to matter greatly. To explore the ways that interactions matter requires a common vocabulary and understanding of key concepts, such as the notion of a "social network" and relevant concepts that have emerged from the social networks literature. We then can survey a range of specific interpersonal communication behaviors, each of which relates in some way to the notion of sharing information. Having those various concepts in hand will be useful for our subsequent discussion and can enrich understanding of the panoply of interpersonal engagement options available now in the 21st century.

Social Networks and Relevant Principles

Castells[1] defined a network simply as a set of interconnected nodes, open to expansion but nonetheless characterized by the proximity of nodes to one another relative to all other nodes at a similar level of conceptual organization. A node can be virtually any unit that can be characterized as somehow being linked or not to another similar unit. Countries connected by economic exchanges, organizations linked by contractual agreements, or neurons connected by synapses are all examples of nodes. Our discussion will focus on individuals as nodes that can be connected by formal or informal relationships with others. For example, a group of college students belonging to the same sorority may constitute a social network, as could residents of city block, or members of the same mosque, or a geographically dispersed group of friends connected to one another through social media sites such as Facebook, Google+, or Pinterest.

Members in a network may share a single point of connection. But, importantly, individual members of a social network also will be more or less connected to other members of the network. It would stretch credibility to discuss "the Latino population in the United States" as a coherent social network, for example, just as it would be a mistake to describe "local television news viewers" in that way. In the former case, demographic labels alone do not guarantee connections between members or even any single hub. In the latter case, individual television stations garner audiences, each of which may be considered a network but which together do not offer a sufficient shared focus to argue for a collective.

Arguably, social networks are a (if not the) fundamental organizational structure for society, as the central governing constraints of physical place have been supplanted at least to some extent by information as the key ingredient for social organization. Castells[1] stated that the "flows of messages and images between networks constitute the basic thread of our social structure" (p. 508). While this shift toward a networked society undoubtedly has made some collective endeavors more efficient—as groups can leverage the collective experience of many members rather than reinventing wheels in each locality—a society characterized by networks is still vulnerable to the development of distinct tiers of existence, planes of interpersonal exchanges that are productive but that typically do not intersect.

The social network concept has been in vogue in recent years as an explanation for human behavior. Bobashev and Anthony,[2] for example, found that demographic factors describing categories of individuals did not fully account for marijuana trial and concluded instead that drug use appears to be a function of social clustering. More recently, Christakis and Fowler[3] described network clustering of everything from obesity to suicide to the experience of happiness.

For decades, scholars have observed social clustering and hypothesized that ties between people can help to explain sociological phenomena. Lessons learned from those observations directly inform expectations for group differences and inequality in information sharing. For example, we can find support not only for the idea that interpersonal relationships can offer a bridge for information flow but also for the notion that the characteristics of social networks facilitate or hinder such flow among groups of people. Several decades ago, for instance, Granovetter[4] pointed to the crucial importance of what he calls weak ties *between* networks of people in explaining the likelihood of success in finding a job: over and above family or close friend relations, less intimate acquaintances appear to have been crucial in helping people locate new employment. Granovetter's emphasis on weak ties as an information resource fosters the roots of a central premise for our present discussion: without bridging connections between networks as vital pathways for information, all that remains are separate network islands on which people essentially do not enjoy interpersonal exchange with any acquaintances outside of their network.

Brown and Reingen[5] later added evidence relevant to the importance of having access to well-connected people by studying the everyday process of locating a piano teacher, a process that often involves word-of-mouth referrals rather than response to large-scale advertising campaigns. They found that people other than family, friends, or neighbors typically serve as bridges between small groups of people. In other words, when tracing the path of referrals person by person back to the original music teacher, relatively weak ties that happened to exist helped to explain how a teacher well known in one group became known to another group. Without such a weak tie bridge, some groups would not have had access to the same music education resources.

The internal structure of social groups also can affect their vulnerability to external sources of information. Moody and White,[6] for example, focused on what they call the structural cohesion of groups—the extent of interconnection between multiple members of a group—in trying to understand the evolution of opinions within the group over time. They noted that the extent to which a group includes multiple relationships between members makes it less vulnerable to domination by a single outside force or to easy dissolution. Conversely, some groups are relatively dependent on a single link to a source outside the group.

Empirical description of the shape and structure of networks also forecasts disparity between individuals in their ability and likelihood to enjoy links with others. Scholars have observed that distribution of connections (or links) among network hubs (or nodes) tends not to be uniformly distributed but actually tends toward what has been called a power law distribution.[7] In other words, most linkages in a system tend to run through a small number of hubs rather than more proportionate distribution.

This tendency is at work in discussions that unfold online. If we conceptualize online conversations as networks of commentators and respondents—such as the asynchronous sequence of exchanges found in response to a news story on a media outlet website—then we should see a heterogeneous configuration in conversational exchanges as well, such that some posts will attract more responses than others. Himelboim[8] applied this general pattern adeptly to hypothesize that online discussion boards, with their threads of postings from users in response to an initially posted question or comment, would illustrate this pattern. Leveraging access to archival online discussion group data from Microsoft, he analyzed Usenet conversation threads over a 5-year period and found that a small group of individuals in these groups attracted a disproportionately large number of replies and different replying authors.

We also can find the roots of other relevant hypotheses in the network literature. While weak ties appear to be important, strong ties also have a place in our discussion. In fact, even considering what makes a tie weak or strong yields ideas about the type of information that people will share with friends and the possibilities for reciprocal information sharing over time. For example, Granovetter's early operational definition of the "strength" of an interpersonal tie is illuminating as a conceptual starting place. Granovetter[4] reasonably argued that we define the strength of a tie as a combination of the "amount of time, the emotional intensity, the intimacy (mutual confiding), and the reciprocal services which characterize the tie" (p. 1361). This insightful description emphasizes the existence of relationships across time, of shared feeling between two people that can extend beyond simple logic, and of the importance of mutual acknowledgment in relationship maintenance. The possibility for relationship evolution and change, the motivating force of emotional arousal, and the allowance for two-way information flow all forecast important elements of the account of interpersonal interaction that features prominently in this book.

Recognition of our humanity—not only our social selves, but also our susceptibility to emotion, our tendency to learn from role models, and our earnest quests—will help us to step beyond social network accounts. The substantial empirical utility of social networks as a predictor of human behavior does not offer all the insight needed to forecast why people will or will not spread, reinforce, or quell information. Much of the observational work describing network clustering of behavior does not, for example, necessarily focus on the specific *manner* in which individuals interact with each other. One can describe the tendency of network A to permit risky sexual behavior relative to network B without understanding the myriad ways that permission is granted or communicated. Data showing the clustering of positive perceptions of such behavior may not shed light on exactly how information about that behavior is shared, whether in the form of a wink, a verbal invitation, or a response to a Twitter post.

A catalogue of information-sharing behavior will be useful to account for why people do or do not tend to pass along information about health, well-being, and how the universe appears to work. How is it that we interact with other people to somehow share information? Let us count the ways. Each of the following sections describes a distinct behavior or phenomenon relevant to the broad concept of information sharing. Figure 1 depicts many of these examples.

Figure 1. Example information-sharing behaviors

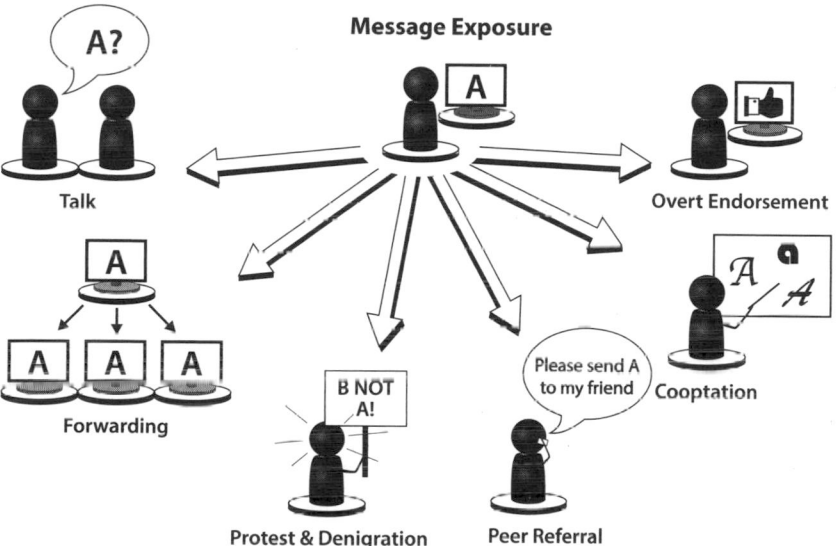

Note: The letters "A" and "B" represent messages. *Talk* refers to verbal expression by two or more mutually co-oriented people, which can occur face-to-face or via telephone or computer. *Forwarding* refers to a person redirecting a copy of an e-mail or other information she or he receives to another person. *Protest & Denigration* refers to commentary a person might express to others regarding an original message. *Peer Referral* refers to a person nominating another to receive information, which might also involve direct forwarding of an offer or incentive from an advertising campaign. *Cooptation* refers to adaptation of a message to create a revised or new message. *Overt Endorsement* refers to explicit acknowledgment that a person approves a message, such as "liking" a post on Facebook.

Conversation (or Talk)

The image of two people engaged in conversation, perhaps at an office water cooler or gathered in a barbershop or while sitting on the front steps of a building, is what many people likely envision when they think about news, rumors, or other information spreading by word of mouth. The very mundane nature of such experience suggests why we also may take the phenomenon for granted, both overestimating the extent to which everyone experiences conversation equally and overlooking the complexity of interaction that occurs regularly in our midst.

Attempting to define conversation is a useful exercise. In earlier work,[9] Marco Yzer and I struggled with precisely this challenge as we attempted to outline specific roles that conversation might play in explaining mass media campaign effects on everything from voting behavior to condom use. We concluded that conversation is fundamentally an observable *behavioral* phenomenon involving multiple people constrained by human motivations and skills, and with important consequences, an observation that is a useful starting point for our discussion.

Social interaction scholars offer helpful assistance when trying to label most people's everyday experiences. Cappella,[10] for example, noted that interaction occurs when person A's trajectory of behavior is influenced by person B over and above what we would expect person A to do based on what person A had been doing up until that point. In other words, to claim that the two had a meaningful interaction, person B needs to be somehow responsible for slowing, accelerating, or modifying person A's actions. Conversation, as an interaction involving words in some way, also would require two or more people verbally interacting. Considered in that way, one-way monologues, not unlike those some of us may have endured on an awful blind date, might be less ideal as an interaction example than a conversation in which one person acknowledges and addresses their words to another person who also is engaged. Even more extreme is the example of a televised speech from the surgeon general on the importance of avoiding trans fats, which would not likely qualify as interaction in this sense because broadcast television content (at least once planned) occurs whether or not anyone specific is sitting in their living room watching, let alone responding directly back to the broadcast source.

In light of these ideas, the phenomenon of conversation needs to involve *mutually co-oriented* participants and that such interaction can affect participants' choices for subsequent actions.[11,12] Of course, not every conversation necessarily will persuade or change one of the participant's minds. Some conversation is mundane and part of everyday routine, such as a brief exchange in the elevator. Nonetheless, as interaction between mutually co-oriented people, every conversation has the potential to reinforce existing beliefs, to remind a person of perceptions or ideas, or even to introduce new information. Additionally, reinforced or introduced ideas can affect future behavior.

On a simple level, conversation offers a forum in which information from other sources can be repeated and in which people may get exposed to new information. Returning to the water cooler example for a moment, imagine that one coworker is telling another about a new lactose-free pizza recipe she used to make dinner the night before. The coworker might have seen the recipe on a morning television news show; repeating the recipe at the water cooler may result in another person learning about it for the first time. The story gets even more interesting if we consider conversation to be a dance of sorts between multiple actors. As such, conversation is likely to be influenced by an array of factors related to human needs and desires as well as constraints that involve the place or setting in which the conversation occurs.[13-18] A conversation at the water cooler might have involved lactose-free pizza because the relatively public venue, with others walking by, hampered the willingness of the duo to discuss more dramatic information about a scandal at the office or family relationships.

Consequently, conversations involve more than just simple information delivery that has been planned in advance. As behavior with the potential for impact on social relationships, conversations often do not go as initially planned because people respond to evolving circumstances as conversations unfold.[19] A planned conversation about the need to practice safer sexual behavior may end up, after a variety of twists and turns, in a teary argument and late-night drama. A planned talk about the need for one's friend to eat more or to see a doctor about potential anorexia may end up in someone slamming a locker door. An anticipated conversation about recycling rules in one's new town may get diverted into a consideration of what colors to paint the walls of a newly purchased house. Conversation, in other words, is not always an efficient tool for persuasion; sometimes it is a messy interaction that introduces complication and consternation.

Forwarding

Not all interpersonal interaction involves a face-to-face exchange. Imagine that a man reads in the local morning newspaper a compelling account of why men 50 years or older should be screened for colorectal cancer. Decades ago, that man might have photocopied the article and put copies in the mailboxes of his friends at work. Today, he might forward the electronic version of the story to coworkers via e-mail or he might post a link to the story on a social media site. Consider the example of a photograph posted and reposted across a network of people through Facebook or the example of a celebrity Tweet subsequently retweeted by thousands of people via Twitter.

One friend forwarding information to another friend presents a clear example of how social connections could operate in the spread of information about health and science. Starbird and Palen[20] looked at two natural disasters in which people used Twitter to forward information: responses to the spring 2009 flooding of the Red River in North Dakota and Minnesota, and the 2009 grassfires that plagued Oklahoma. This study identified a tendency for Twitter users who lived near those events to retweet, or forward wholesale, information originally posted by mass media organizations about the changing conditions and related emergency response.

As a departure from the archetypal example of conversation on the front steps of a building, the examples of forwarded photocopies or retweeted headlines highlight a conceptual dilemma, namely, does an interaction have to occur face-to-face to draw our consideration? Decades of early research on interpersonal communication centered on face-to-face interaction, yet now, interpersonal scholars agree that such communication can occur in a variety of settings and in a variety of ways.[21] Similarly, our catalogue of information-sharing behavior also should include more than just face-to-face exchanges.

Similar to the case of television, changes in information technology in the past two decades have made it possible for an extended exchange to occur between two people who are not physically in the same place or even in sync in the timing. Such a change has invited a wide range of communication research that primarily involves so-called computer-mediated exchanges between people,[22-24] which is not to say that everyone believes such exchanges are as efficient or satisfying as face-to-face interaction. Following her study of numerous online chat streams, Herring[25] concluded that online chat, one example of online communication, is often incoherent and disjointed. Nonetheless, Internet-based exchanges of text posts may be gradually more acceptable over time. Almost 10 years ago, Baym and colleagues[26] already had reported that college students perceived Internet-based conversation as only slightly lower in quality than face-to-face interaction. Moreover, Papacharissi[27] made a similar point in her review of online interaction scholarship, claiming that both online and face-to-face interactions reflect human needs and desires and consequently are not necessarily distinct.

Overt Endorsement

For a number of years, contemporary Facebook users have had the option to click on a thumbs up icon as a way of responding to information posted by someone else in their social network. Google+ users can add a "+1" to a post as a way of signaling their approval. Such an act is seemingly innocuous and both its ease and subtlety likely contribute to its appeal. Nonetheless, any review of information-sharing behavior would be incomplete to not mention such acts of overt endorsement. In fact, a number of public health campaigns appear to encourage such endorsement as a major focus of their efforts. The US Department of Health and Human Services, for example, launched a Facebook application in 2010 that allowed users to declare "I'm a flu fighter" and to announce their flu vaccination status to all friends to whom they are connected through the site.

Users of social media sites that allow for peer indication of approval offer opportunities for immediate feedback on one's pronouncements and comments from a social network. Conceptually, the mere opportunity for immediate feedback from a geographically dispersed network of contacts offers a step for additional interpersonal back-and-forth that is somewhat distinct from the earlier example of the photocopy about cancer screening distributed to office mailboxes. The absence or abundance of electronic approval one receives in response to a post may encourage or discourage similar posts in the future. Also, the simple count of endorsements that a particular statement or content receives may be processed by anyone viewing the content as an indication of prominent social norms. These norms are consequential, both in terms of the number of people who engage in a particular behavior and the beliefs that others have about whether one ought to perform a behavior. Additionally, the perceptions of norms, or what others think, often predict human behavior over and above what a person otherwise thinks about a behavior.[28]

The ease and simplicity afforded by electronic tools for social interaction do not guarantee depth or richness in interaction. In that regard, use of overt endorsement applications, such as star ratings on an online restaurant review site, differ qualitatively from in-depth conversation that two people might conduct. In fact, such endorsement tools arguably have made social interaction shallower and more formulaic among those who use them. Carr[29] suggested that online interaction tools offer "scripts" that "mechanize the messy processes of intellectual exploration and even social attachment" (p. 218). As we flit from alert to alert regarding friends' updates and endorsements of our comments, "the Net reroutes our vital paths and diminishes our capacity for contemplation … altering the depth of our emotions as well as our thoughts" (p. 221). At the same time, it also may be the case that such shallow interaction sufficiently lowers the bar as to invite a wider range of participants than more challenging forms of social interaction.

Commentary and Cooptation

Revisiting the earlier example of the man sharing the newspaper article on colorectal cancer screening, one might imagine that same man writes in the margins of the photocopied story a lighthearted disclaimer that he does not want to be the "butt of jokes" for passing the story along. In this example, the content that actually reaches people is a hybrid. Clearly, it contains the original material but also carries the commentary of the person passing it along.

More complex examples abound. Current technology allows teenagers the ability to sample music and video, add their own content, and to post hybrid content for friends to see. Some individuals have even gone further to take prominent pieces of existing content and to weave them together into an artistic "mash-up." One example that garnered hundreds of thousands of views following its initial posting featured a conglomerate that seamlessly melded old footage from videos by the singer Madonna and by the British band The Sex Pistols. Such hybrid pastiches of content beg the question of what counts as simple diffusion and what needs to be labeled as adaptation, transformation, and evolution of information as a result of individuals using material to communicate with one another.

Given the plethora of content relevant to health behavior available in popular culture, such cooptation offers individuals the chance to further disseminate bits and pieces of relevant information. Imagine a mash-up including one of myriad hip-hop or country references to brands of alcohol. Nonetheless, the opportunity also offers a chance for people to potentially undermine the original intent of the material. Well-intentioned campaigns may provide fodder for their own mockery. For example, Massachusetts and Florida, among other states, have focused some campaign efforts on the characterization of tobacco as "stinky" and "smelly" and "gross." Anecdotal evidence suggests that at least some teens have co-opted the language and ironically embraced it as a way of mocking the anti-tobacco effort.

Referral

Social connections can direct information even without direct contact. Consider the various opportunities people now have to nominate others to receive the same information as they have or to participate in the same program that they themselves have done. Examples are everywhere. SolarCity, one of the largest solar panel installers in the United States, offered current customers a cash incentive for referrals of other people who would like to have panels installed. Carolina Donor Services, an organ donation organization in North Carolina, offered people the chance to Refer-A-Friend and recommend that someone they know to be invited to consider organ donation. ViaCord, a cord blood banking organization in Massachusetts, offered people financial incentives to recruit their friends to donate umbilical cord blood (and stem cells) from their newborn babies. In an example that we will explore in more depth later, the Minnesota Department of Health offered underinsured cancer screening participants who have benefited from a free screening program a chance to refer a friend to the same program.

Peer-referral programs offer opportunities for participants to ensure that their friends and family members have access to the same programs as they do. However, this type of referral does not necessarily ensure universal access across all people in a population. Access to information in these cases is affected to some extent by one's connection to the person making the referral.

Theoretical Comparison of Information-Sharing Behaviors

Information-sharing behaviors differ in at least two theoretically important ways: the extent of physical interaction permitted or encouraged and the affordance of social presence. In short, some forms of information sharing do not encourage lengthy exchanges and some forms of sharing behaviors yield relatively less of a sense of physical intimacy with another person.

First, the scope of likely interaction with another person, in terms of time and content, varies across our catalogue of sharing possibilities. A conversation, at least theoretically, could last for minutes or hours and could involve multiple exchanges between partners over an extended period. Simply forwarding an e-mail to a family member without any additional commentary is, compared with a lengthy conversation, a relatively quick act (though reading the forwarded material may take a while). Clandestinely signing up a friend to receive material in the mail from an organization might not even involve any direct interaction between the instigator and the friend at all.

Second, and on a related plane, the information-sharing behaviors likely vary in the extent to which they afford social presence. Lee[30] reviewed the development of thinking about presence as it relates to communication behavior in general and with regard to electronically mediated contexts, such as watching a video or being immersed in a multiplayer virtual reality game. Presence, according to Lee, is "a psychological state in which the virtuality of experience is unnoticed" (p. 32). In other words, full presence occurs when a person experiences a context without any indication of the artificiality of that context. Artificiality itself may be experienced or understood differently by different people. Nonetheless, Lee is interested in the experience of a person walking along an actual street in her or his neighborhood relative to watching a slide show of a person walking down a virtual representation of that street. Importantly, Lee then focused special attention on the social dimension of presence and defines the experience with reference to human interaction. A face-to-face conversation in which both people are bodily in the same room would exemplify social presence; a chat using a Facebook application in which both parties type on computers while sitting thousands of miles apart would hold relatively less potential for social presence. This is not to say that a computer-based interaction cannot be emotionally evocative and intellectually stimulating. An electronically mediated experience with lower social presence need not, from this perspective, rule out meaningful interaction altogether. Moreover, sitting face-to-face with someone need not guarantee a satisfying communication experience, to which many of us can attest.

Acknowledging at least general differences in the amount of interaction and the social presence possibilities of these various sharing behaviors highlights subtle differences in the types of sharing that each behavior affords. As Cortese and Seo[31] posited, and supported with some evidence, computer-mediated interaction may actually encourage greater disclosure of opinions and otherwise uncomfortable revelation even if the sheer amount (or time) of interaction is curtailed by two people not being face-to-face. For our discussion, the acknowledgment of differences in these information-sharing behaviors suggests two important ideas. First, these behaviors, while conceptually related, are not completely interchangeable. Consequently, we will need to draw on examples beyond a simple, face-to-face talk throughout our discussion, even if such a conversation is a convenient archetype. The reasons why people do not share information when talking with others may not be the same reasons why people do not post information to a social media site, for example. So we will need a broad lens to capture reasons for disparities across those differing contexts. Second, noticing these subtle but theoretically noteworthy differences across this range of information-sharing behaviors also might suggest potential remedies, if such remedies to disparity are sought. Consequently, facilitation of certain types of information sharing may help, even if little can be done to overcome the difficulties of other types of information sharing.

Summary

Information sharing occurs not only in face-to-face conversations but also across a range of behaviors. Some of those behaviors are facilitated by emergent technologies; some have been with us for a long time. While there are nuanced and noteworthy differences between these various behaviors, based even on everyday experience we also can predict that people vary in their tendency to engage each other, particularly with regard to specialized topics. It is important to note that the mere fact of information sharing between people does not guarantee the veracity or quality of the information being shared. Rumors certainly abound, for example, largely through peer-to-peer sharing. Nonetheless, if we are concerned with the spread of information about human health and well-being or about important developments in any of a variety of sciences, then variance between people in any of the information-sharing behaviors presented in this chapter has potential consequence, especially if people vary for reasons of avoidable social disadvantage.

To further build a case for caring about differences in information-sharing behaviors, we next need to better understand why they arise. So the next few chapters examine the evidence regarding the origins of information-sharing differences that signal various factors that may offer some explanations.

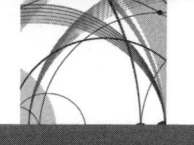

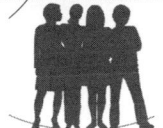

CHAPTER 4

Who One Is Matters:
Individual-Level Factors That
Affect Sharing

Each of the next three chapters presents a set of factors that help to explain why information about science and health is not universally and uniformly discussed. Each chapter examines a different level of analysis for factors that affect information sharing: individual-level factors, community-level factors, and content-level factors. To illustrate the shifts from one level to another, it is helpful to consider a single example from each of the three perspectives.

In fall 2012, the eastern United States witnessed the arrival of Hurricane Sandy, a major storm that caused extensive flooding in New York, New Jersey, and elsewhere. The magnitude of the storm led some observers to wonder if the event was a harbinger of future disasters.[1] The story of Sandy offered a number of different reporting angles and subsequent discussion focused specifically on scientific research, including consideration of electric grid vulnerabilities in the United States, investigation of water-related issues, and scientific research on climate change and storms. In the days following landfall of the storm, however, the most mentioned topics on the social media site Twitter clearly were not all related to the storm, as popular topics included Halloween and the Disney company's purchase of the *Star Wars* franchise.[*] To help organize our discussion, we need to ask a key question: Why was that?

Consider the science behind Hurricane Sandy as the example for the next three chapters. One set of factors that helps to explain why some people spent late October talking with others or sharing information with others about scientific research on hurricanes involves individual demographic, psychological, and socioeconomic differences. This chapter focuses on variables that describe an individual person. People vary in myriad ways: they can be tall or short, more or less novelty-seeking, or richer or poorer. Some of those differences should predict a person's tendency to share information with others about a topic such as climate research related to storms.

---

[*] A look at http://twitter.com, accessed October 31, 2012, offered evidence of posting trends.

The literature on health disparities and on gaps in understanding of science suggests wide discrepancies between individuals in what they know about health and science.[2,3] Such discrepancies appear to be a function of both information exposure and information-seeking behavior, among other factors. Oelschlegel and colleagues,[4] for example, studied telephone call logs for a free health information service in Tennessee. Despite efforts to provide the program to all local residents free of charge, the study found a major discrepancy in the use of the system based on socioeconomic status: most of the calls came from relatively advantaged ZIP Codes, whereas only a minority of calls came from ZIP Codes with more than 10 percent of residents living below the poverty level. This pattern suggests that information gaps are enduring.

The gaps between people in knowledge about health, medicine, and other science research suggest that people hold different conceptual models of well-being, health behavior, and the natural world. (Whether the simple fact of discrepancies in factual knowledge is something to bemoan is a matter of important debate.[5]) In light of these knowledge differences, it is not surprising to predict that people also will vary in their tendency to talk to and share information with their friends, family members, and neighbors. But exactly which individual-level factors matter? In other words, what explains why it is that some people actively engage with their peers on certain topics and others do not?

Scholars have pursued the question of exactly who shares information with others for decades. At least two classic mass communication effect studies— Katz and Lazarsfeld's[6] early assessment of interpersonal communication as a mediator of mass media effects on individuals' opinions and an investigation by Rogers[7] of the so-called diffusion of innovations—highlighted the notion that not everyone is equally popular as an information hub. Both of these studies attempted to describe people as being more or less likely to adopt particular information, beliefs, or innovations and as being more or less likely to serve as bridging hubs (called "opinion leaders") through which information is disseminated to others in their social networks. Whereas these early studies identified the fact of our networked structure (as Katz and Lazarsfeld noted) or the notion that people are "early" or "late" adopters (as Rogers noted), we nonetheless have lacked a complete answer as to who is more or less likely to share information, especially regarding topics such as health and scientific research.

Importantly, knowing who might serve as an information hub alone will not offer a complete story of information diffusion through a system. We also will need to know something about the nature of networks surrounding a person, for example, as discussed in Chapter 5. Nonetheless, identifying reasons why people may vary in their likelihood of interpersonal engagement with regard to various topics will begin to explain why we can expect health and science knowledge disparities between groups of people.

We can start with demographic description. In a nutshell, individuals of different socioeconomic status or educational background appear to share health and science information to a different extent and in different ways. Such differences likely mask more interesting patterns, so it is important to be careful in causal attribution. Why some individuals reach out to others and other individuals do not reach out is not entirely an inherent function of social status; it is also a function of learned skills and even biological tendency.

Socioeconomic Status

Limited evidence suggests that socioeconomic resources may facilitate greater likelihood of sharing certain types of information. An example from a state-level effort to prompt peer information sharing is illustrative. For a number of years, the Minnesota Department of Health has made free mammograms available to uninsured and underinsured women. More importantly, the health department also attempted to advertise this program through a "Refer a Friend" effort that allowed women to nominate their friends and family to receive notice of the offer. Colleagues and I[8] studied who exactly, among a sample of thousands of women, took advantage of the opportunity to pass mammography information along to family and friends. The findings showed that socioeconomic status, among other factors, predicted information sharing.

The study results are noteworthy for two reasons. First, most people who were offered the opportunity to refer others to get the same benefit as what they received initially did not opt to refer anyone. The majority of participants nominated no one they knew to receive information about the program. Second, the pattern of referral suggested a socioeconomic divide in the extent to which participants referred other people. Both income level and having at least some form of insurance positively predicted, at a bivariate level, the number of peer nominations a woman provided.

In a final model that included a variety of predictors, insurance status continued to predict nomination. Women who already benefited from some form of insurance (even though technically they were still underinsured) were the women who were passing along the benefit of free mammograms to others, not necessarily women in the state who had no health insurance at all.

Individuals who were (relatively) advantaged were the most active in sharing information. Perhaps these women knew contact information for more other women than did uninsured participants. Perhaps insured women tended to better comprehend—or be in a position to realize—the benefits of screening. Perhaps insured women thought it was more likely that their friends and family would be able to take advantage of the opportunity. Regardless of the reason, at least one indicator of socioeconomic status was associated with peer nomination, which is evidence that differences in social standing are related to information-sharing differences.

Education

Arguably, people with higher levels of (formal) education tend to talk more about certain topics than other people, particularly with regard to environmental science or innovations in medical research. Additionally, the more education people have, all other factors being equal, the more likely they are to be familiar with a wide range of research and public policy issues. Consequently, in trying to understand information diffusion, one might argue that two people who vary in education may also differ in their likelihood to share with others science or health information that they may encounter, especially with regard to technical information or policy-related facts.

Data from Tanzania, for example, suggest that individuals with less education are relatively less likely to be sought out for conversation about family planning and HIV prevention than those with more education. After studying people who listened to a radio soap opera that dealt with sexual health issues, Mohammed[9] concluded that people in Tanzania tended to seek out and engage conversational partners at equal or higher levels of education when discussing family planning or HIV prevention. Such a pattern suggests conversational network homogeneity in terms of who talks with whom about crucially important health topics. It also suggests disjuncture in interpersonal information flow as a function of educational differences.

A study conducted by graduate students at the University of Minnesota offers another illustrative example. This study proposed and tested a hypothesis focused on educational disparity, namely, that individuals who differ in educational attainment also would differ in the extent to which seeing television content on relatively specialized topics, such as climate change or transportation safety, would prompt them to later talk with other people about those topics.[10]

Researchers recruited a group of adults and then experimentally assigned some participants to see television news segments in which they had embedded short announcements on global warming and transportation safety. In a control group, participants saw the same news segment but without the embedded announcements and with commercial advertisements in their place. At follow-up (at least a week after seeing the original news program), researchers surveyed participants about their interactions with family and friends during the time since they engaged the first part of the study.

The study suggested support for the contention that education matters: seeing the inserted global warming and transportation safety announcements only predicted later talk among participants who were well educated. In general, participants who saw the announcements were not any more likely than those who did not see the announcements to subsequently talk about global warming or transportation safety. Among the more educated participants in the study, seeing the television content in question did predict subsequent talk. That pattern was exactly what was hypothesized to occur. More specifically, educational attainment and experimentally assigned exposure interacted to predict subsequent relevant conversation ($p < .05$).

A variety of mechanisms could explain the impact of education, including the tendency of individuals with more education to hold more extensive preexisting cognitive schema with regard to public policy issues, such as global warming and transportation safety; greater confidence among those who are well educated; and the potential impact of alienation related to social stratification among those who are less educated. Individuals with an extensive preexisting cognitive framework regarding public policy, for example, likely held more mental material that was vulnerable to activation through exposure to the experimental stimulus and perhaps were more likely to retain information from that content over a long enough period to later engage in relevant conversation using that knowledge. On a different plane, perhaps individuals who are well educated have greater confidence or self-efficacy in initiating conversations. That possibility will arise again in a later section of this chapter.

These results also may reflect important aspects of social stratification, alienation, and information engagement. Individuals who perceive themselves to be (or who structurally are) in positions of relative disadvantage often tend to demonstrate less information gain than their counterparts.[11] Importantly, such differential information gain seems to be a function of alienation or perceived powerlessness, suggesting that another factor driving information disengagement is the perceived lack of information utility. Motivation, in other words, also matters. Participants who are less educated may well have viewed both initial topical learning and the prospect of talking with others about such information later as relatively useless given their own perceived or real lack of authority to actually direct or encourage any societal change.

Perceived Topical Relevance

Interpersonal communication scholars have long pointed to the importance of perceived relevance in predicting people's interaction. In short, people tend to talk more frequently about topics that they believe to be personally relevant or important to them.[12,13] For any given message, individuals for whom it is most relevant (or those who know people for whom the message is relevant) are likely to be the ones who make the effort to talk about the information with anyone else. Consequently, perception of relevance is at least partly a function of the frequency of past thinking about a topic.

Sehulster[13] explained this tendency by pointing to the cognitive structure of the human brain. Because we actively draw from memory when participating in conversation, we typically find it relatively easy to discuss topics that have been frequently engaged in the past because those topics occupy prominent and well-worn cognitive spaces. When stimuli linked to a topic appear on television or on a website, for example, conversation about the topic in question is relatively easy and convenient. When a topic is chronically salient, fodder for related conversation will be at the tip of one's tongue. A set of friends who are all basketball fans and gathered at a bar watching television should be more likely to engage one another in conversation when a television news story about last night's game is shown than when a story appears regarding drought in a faraway region of the world, all other factors being equal.

This example also points out that *where* one is (in terms of situation) helps to determine what one might consider most relevant. Wagner[14] pointed out that people do not live in a single, uniform world but instead regularly transition between different planes and contexts. Each of those contexts carries particular constraints and opportunities for social interaction. People may operate in professional arenas using specialized language and knowledge and then in the same day move to other contexts, such as talking with a cashier at the pharmacy or calling a spouse on the telephone to arrange dinner. Nonetheless, many people often have daily routines, or chronic access to a set of particular contexts, that differentiate them from others and consistently invite certain types of information sharing.

Perceived Understanding

Logic and evidence suggest that people will be most active in sharing information with others in instances in which those sharing the information grasp the gist of the content and those with whom the information is being sharing are capable of understanding it. If we assume that most people are at least somewhat cautious in their everyday engagement with others and that they tend not to venture far beyond conversational topics they believe they comprehend, then another constraint on information sharing is a person's perceived understanding of the topic of the information in question.

For instance, think back to a Thanksgiving dinner you celebrated with a large gathering of family, friends, or even strangers. At least some of the conversation likely focused on the food on the table, a shared point of focus for everyone. Beyond that, chances are that most of the conversation that unfolded was constrained by the extent to which people around the table understood what was being discussed at least well enough to ask questions or to offer their own commentary. Conversations about particle physics probably only occurred in those dining rooms in which at least two people felt they knew some key concepts or terminology. Science, as an overarching topic, can be daunting for those who think that people like themselves cannot understand it sufficiently to discuss it. Many people will avoid such conversation if they feel ill-prepared

This rationale suggests that in any group of people there are distinct differences in tendency to talk with others about science (including human health research), technology, engineering, or mathematics that stem directly from perceived understanding. It should be noted that perceived understanding, as a motivating force, probably persists regardless of whether a person actually understands the material in question from an objective perspective. For example, we have all probably had the experience of encountering a person who is more than willing to chat about a topic on which their factual knowledge is suspect.

Alicia Torres of the American Institute of Physics and I, with the assistance of the National Science Foundation, investigated the hypothesis that perceived understanding of science will predict talk about the role of scientists and science in everyday life.[15] We conducted an experiment in which some people were essentially taught about a variety of science topics and encouraged to consider science and mathematics as being topics that people like them can understand. We then assessed whether later they were more likely than they had been previously to talk about such topics with those in their social network.

We studied a cross-section of the adult television news audience. Participants in this study ranged from 18 to 90 years old; average (or mean) age in the sample was 51. People from a variety of racial and ethnic backgrounds participated, including people self-identifying as white or Caucasian, African American, Latino (or Latina), and a variety of other racial and ethnic backgrounds. A little more than half (or 53 percent) of the participants were female. Educational attainment also varied, with 40 percent of the participants having completed at least a 4-year undergraduate degree and 60 percent reported some college or less. The study specifically recruited individuals who lived in the Buffalo, New York, Designated Market Area (meaning the 10 counties surrounding and including Buffalo that comprise the television market in that area) to participate in the study. None of the American Institute of Physics news stories currently were running in that market, which offered a relatively clean slate and made the area a useful one for the study.

Rather than conducting a laboratory study, this research assessed people's activity in their own homes and neighborhoods. We mailed participants experimental materials that consisted of an explanatory letter and either a DVD or a VHS tape (depending on preference and technology access) containing 7 days of the programming and then followed up with each participant by telephone after the week of viewing. We randomly assigned people who signed up for the study either to see some of the news stories in question or not. In two different experimental treatment conditions, people viewed science stories embedded in a week's worth of television news programming. One group saw more of the stories than the other group, although both saw at least some stories during the week. In the control (or comparison) group, participants were invited to watch the same week's worth of television news without any of the science stories; instead they saw unrelated general interest stories where the science stories would have been.

The results revealed that showing people the science news stories in question not only raised their confidence relative to others but also prompted them to talk more. Randomly assigned science news exposure predicted simple group differences in perceived understanding of science and talk about science. A comparison of the full treatment condition to the control revealed significant mean differences for both perceived understanding and post-exposure science talk.

The findings also showed a moderate bivariate relationship between perceived understanding and talk (Pearson's $r = .22$, $p < .01$) that persisted as a significant relationship even after controlling for other factors. Perceived understanding of science and math was not the only factor predicting subsequent talk. Whether a person tended to have such conversations in the past significantly contributed to the final predictive model, as did simply having seen the news stories (regardless of a specific boost in perceived understanding). Nonetheless, the results suggest a link between perceived ability to understand and conversation about science that existed over and above the effects of education, current job status, and conversational history. Together, this suggests that bolstering confidence may offer a route to overcome some of the socioeconomic and education-based differences in information sharing discussed earlier. This idea will return again in Chapter 8.

We can find more evidence for a relationship between perceived topical knowledge and tendency to talk about a topic with data in a more recent national survey of Americans' perceptions of energy.[16] In that work, we posited that energy information sharing across various modalities, such as posting to Facebook or having face-to-face conversations, is a function of objective knowledge, perceived understanding, and other variables. The study measured objective knowledge with an 11-item energy knowledge index developed in consultation with the US Department of Energy and a researcher at Clarkson University. It also measured agreement that energy is a topic that people like the respondent can understand as well as other key variables. The final model demonstrated that perceived understanding predicts information sharing, even over and above objective knowledge and other factors such as education level and age.

What, then, distinguishes people who talk about science or technology from those who do not? Perceived topical understanding is clearly one useful predictor. Over and above factors such as educational background, the nature of a person's employment, and even how much a person specifically knows about a topic, perceived understanding continues to predict talk. A person's sense that they can grasp a particular topic seems to encourage them to pursue interaction with others on that topic. While there is likely some degree of reciprocity in the relationship (as one might learn over time that they can understand a topic by being exposed to conversations about that topic), it also seems likely that confidence affects information sharing.

Personality

Might personality characteristics predict a person's tendency to share information with others? If so, might one's own likelihood of peer-to-peer information exposure be a function of the types of personalities populating one's network? That biology could be relevant to our discussion may seem to be a leap, but further consideration suggests substantial reason to expect our enduring psychological makeup to predispose us to information sharing, both in terms of giving and receiving.

The quest to characterize opinion leaders or those who tend to be conversational hubs in social networks often invites speculation about the possible importance of inherent differences linked to personality. Katz and Lazarsfeld,[6] for example, posited that "gregariousness" explains opinion leadership, but they also did not articulate an explicit biological or psychological basis for that claim and so the premise risks tautology without further explication. Other scholars have raised the possibility that "personality strength" is something that may differentiate person A from person B and predict conversational tendency.[17] Theoretically, we can go further to look at two personality variables, communication apprehension and sensation seeking, that may affect information sharing in very different ways.

Communication Apprehension and Shyness

In the mid-20th century, academic research on speech performance thrust into the foreground such concepts as stage fright and oral communication anxiety as rhetoricians sought to understand why some people wilted in the spotlight of public speaking opportunities. Pioneers such as James McCroskey led the evolution of the stage fright notion into the more broadly applicable concept of communication apprehension. McCroskey and colleagues largely described communication apprehension as an individual trait. For example, in multiple studies, some people demonstrated anxiety at the prospect of verbal engagement with others and consequently were less likely to talk often with other people.[18-21] The specific anxiousness and reticence that McCroskey identified appears to be a subset of the general shyness that some people experience in everyday life: namely, some people are more reluctant than others to verbally engage their neighbors and colleagues.

The roots of communication apprehension and reticence, as McCroskey and colleagues discovered, appear to be both multifaceted and revealing for this discussion. McCroskey and Richmond,[20] for example, were careful to acknowledge that shyness in general may stem from a lack of conversation skills and may also be a function of anxiety tendencies that are foundationally inherent but also emergent over time as one interacts with the environment in which they live. McCroskey and Richmond[19] also sought to understand why communication apprehension appears to emerge in children from relatively rural areas and found an explanation in the lack of reinforcement and support for the communicatively unsuccessful. For instance, while people growing up in smaller towns may have more opportunities for face-to-face interactions with the same people over time, they also likely have fewer places to turn when their interactions do not go as planned or preferred; consequently, they adjust by learning simply to share less over time.

What can a decades-old program of research inspired by public speaking difficulties tell us about information-sharing disparities? Clearly, some people have different physiological responses to the prospect of engaging others. Over time, those differences can lead to the development of apprehension that appears to suppress at least verbal interaction. This underscores one reason why we should expect inequality in information sharing. However, inequality in apprehension, insofar as it reflects naturally occurring personality diversity, is not as problematic as differences in environmental support available to people over time from an equity perspective. Within that distinction is a foundation for ethical considerations, which Chapter 8 revisits.

Research on oral communication does not necessarily speak directly to prospects for e-mail forwarding, social media posting, or other electronic modalities for information sharing outlined in Chapter 3, so it is also important to consider information sharing outside of face-to-face contexts. Nonetheless, personality-based reticence could impact at least any of the information-sharing modalities that involve direct disclosure of a person's communicative intention, though perhaps not to the same extent. An anxiety-producing conversation is likely more difficult to conduct in person than via text message, for example.

Sensation Seeking

Beyond hindering information sharing, individual differences linked to personality may also facilitate peer-to-peer information diffusion and interpersonal interaction. While anxiety-tendency may suppress one's appetite to interact with others, it is also possible that we can find at least some drivers toward conversation and information sharing in the brain as well. We even might go further and link the tendency to share information with other people with the makeup of the brain. Consider the notion of sensation seeking, a concept that captures at least part of the essence of having an adventurous and curious spirit with which you may or may not relate. Zuckerman[22] offered a succinct view of the characteristic, identifying "sensation seeking" as "the seeking of varied, novel, complex, and intense sensations and experiences, and the willingness to take physical, social, legal, and financial risks for the sake of such experience" (p. 27). The need for sensation manifests itself in myriad risky behaviors, such as bungee jumping, skydiving, driving fast, unsafe sexual behavior, criminal activity, excessive gambling, and too many impulsive purchases.[22-26]

Though the sensation-seeking notion will be useful for our discussion, we also should note a caveat regarding the theoretical concept. Mike Stephenson and I[25] noted that academic observation of sensation seeking may actually mask what in reality are *multiple* neural drivers. In other words, what manifests as sensation seeking may reflect a particular combination of more basic processes. All of us appear to harbor both appetitive and inhibiting systems in our brains. More formally, scholars have labeled these the behavioral approach system (BAS) and behavioral inhibition system (BIS).[27] What sensation-seeking research has done successfully is to focus attention on inherent differences in our appetitive systems; that is, in our tendencies to approach stimuli. Some people need to seek out novel experience and stimulation to reach equilibrium more than others. This observation does not rule out the possibility that people also vary in inhibition, meaning that two people who are equally drawn to novelty—or to stimulating interpersonal interaction—may not be equally likely to actually pursue that stimulating experience because of differences in inhibition.

Nuances regarding underlying concepts aside, general differences in observed sensation-seeking tendency between people seem to be rooted, at least in part, in biochemistry; meaning we can regard sensation seeking as a personality trait based on biological individual differences.[22,28] Biochemical differences between people in terms of dopamine, a chemical tied to the human brain's experience of pleasure, seem to explain sensation seeking.[29,30] Greater tendency to seek sensation is often statistically coincident with lower default levels of dopamine.[25,31] In other words, high-sensation seekers appear to harbor higher optimal levels of stimulation[22,32] essentially because they have lower default levels of dopamine available. Seemingly risky activities provide high-sensation seekers with the extra stimulation they need to achieve their optimal level of physiological arousal, whereas low-sensation seekers need less external stimulation.[31,33]

Although scholars have often considered sensation seeking as a predictor of what some might view as socially unacceptable or at least atypical behaviors, logic suggests the personality trait also should predict general information sharing as well. In fact, Zuckerman[22,34] noted in his foundational reviews of the concept that sociability conventionally has been an aspect of what it means to be a high-sensation seeker. More directly, high- and low-sensation seekers have different conversational tendencies: high sensation seekers talk and seek out others more. Early work[35] on sensation seeking observed that when high-sensation seekers were confined with low-sensation seekers in a room for 8 hours that the high-sensation seekers seemed to talk relatively more. (The question of exactly who would even sign up to sit alone in a room for 8 hours with other study participants, of course, is a compelling query.) In addition, Franken, Gibson, and Mohan[36] found that sensation seeking positively predicted a person's inclination to disclose personal thoughts and feelings to others: high-sensation seekers were more uninhibited and open in their interactions with friends. Why might high-sensation seekers talk more? The potentially stimulating nature of social relationships and conversation offers an explanation. Zuckerman and Link[37] argued that high-sensation seekers needed others primarily as an audience for their performance. Zuckerman[22] also later argued that social relationships are a major source of stimulation and arousal for sensation seekers.

Some recent work directly investigated whether high-sensation seekers are more likely to talk with others about various health or other science topics. David, Cappella, and Fishbein[38] conducted a compelling experiment by encouraging study participants to talk to each other after being shown five different public service announcements regarding marijuana. Participants' relevant conversation was aggregated to measure individuals' total amount of talk about anti-drug messages. By correlating the total talk score with sensation-seeking tendency, this study found that high-sensation seekers talked significantly more than their counterparts. Although this study provides evidence that sensation seeking and talk are statistically related, there is at least one plausible challenge to the hypothesis that personality is the key driver, per se. High-sensation seekers may have been more likely to talk about marijuana (or campaign ads) simply because the topic was more relevant to them or because they had more favorable attitudes toward marijuana. Insofar as high-sensation seekers are more likely to try drugs, as noted earlier, the fact that high-sensation seekers talked more about anti-drug advertisements is not surprising. It suggests an indirect effect of personality, at most. Consequently, we need additional evidence.

More recent evidence goes further to suggest that sensation seeking, over and above the relevance of a topic, predicts talk. Yoori Hwang and I had an opportunity, again with the support of the National Science Foundation and the American Institute of Physics, to study whether sensation seeking predicts how often people talk about science. In short, we found that sensation seeking does forecast one's tendency to engage others in conversation, even when the topic at hand is not directly linked to risky behavior per se.[39]

In addition to a variety of other variables, including the extent to which people talked with others about science, we asked people about their sensation-seeking tendencies. One validated method of assessing sensation seeking, which we used, is to ask people for their agreement with an overall scale comprising items that indicate their interest in, and attraction to, a variety of relatively stimulating or high-risk stimuli. The various items to which respondents reported their agreement included statements such as "I like to do frightening things" and "I like new and exciting experiences, even if I have to break the rules."

In the final data analysis, a number of factors predicted talk with others about science, technology, engineering or mathematics, as one might expect. Higher levels of formal education positively predicted such talk, as did whether or not a person held a science-related job. The extent to which people thought that science and mathematics were topics that someone like them could understand also mattered. Over and above all other factors, though, sensation seeking turned out to be a significant predictor of conversations about science even after controlling for all of the aforementioned and other variables ($p < .01$). Based on these results, inborn and inherited nature, as reflected by one's sensation-seeking tendency, can help explain conversational tendency beyond the simple influence of nurture, that is, learned knowledge or developed interest.

The Limits of Individual Differences

People vary in their likelihood of sharing information, and we have explored numerous reasons in this chapter as to how both demographic factors and personality differences might account for that variation. Individual differences, however, do not explain all aspects of variability in the social diffusion of information or in interpersonal discussion of information. As we will see in the next chapter, individual differences may be more useful in explaining why any two people tend to share information in a particular instance, all other factors being equal, than in accounting for macro-level patterns of societal-level or network-level diffusion. While individual traits and variables are part of the story, where you are, aside from who you are, also appears to play a role, which leads us to examining community-level factors in the next chapter.

CHAPTER 5

Where One Is Matters: Community-Level Factors That Affect Sharing

Let's return to the organizing example from the beginning of Chapter 4: the question of why some people talked about scientific research related to Hurricane Sandy and why some people did not. Chapter 4 outlined the various ways individual characteristics can predispose people to be more or less likely to share information with others. This chapter examines a different level of analysis. What if individuals are constrained, regardless of personality or educational background, by characteristics of the social networks, neighborhood, or community in which they work, play, or live? What if where a person resides, in terms of geographic place or even in terms of your location in time, predicts their access to information or the likelihood of their ability to share information with others?

To extend our exploration of information sharing, we need to focus on variables that describe *communities* of people as they exist in physical places and in online networks. Some neighborhoods are likely better equipped than others to facilitate discussion. Places that had hosted regular community forums on science and public policy or that already were home to lively coffee shops or church basements where people can physically gather, for example, probably witnessed more interaction and information sharing in the days following Hurricane Sandy than did others. We will examine the evidence in this chapter.

From Katz and Lazarsfeld's[1] classic book *Personal Influence* to popular volumes such as Gladwell's[2] *The Tipping Point*, theorists and pundits have posited that a handful of highly influential people can drive the widespread diffusion of information. Beneath that observation, however, is a crucial caveat. Katz[3] himself, in a paper somewhat less well known than the earlier *Personal Influence*, declared that exactly who a person happens to know matters quite a bit in predicting opinion leadership. In an essay celebrating *Personal Influence*, Kadushin[4] also asserted the importance of network availability—either as an active resource or as a latent resource that could potentially be activated—in allowing a person to serve as an information distribution hub and fountain of influence. Relationships and connections between people can lie relatively underutilized, just as other community resources can lie untapped. Snyder and Omoto,[5] for example, noted that even a reservoir of latent altruistic intent can lie dormant without the availability of volunteer organizations and programs that offer formal outlets through which people can sign up to help others. All of this suggests that having a preexisting network infrastructure of some sort in place can be an important precursor to widespread information sharing between people in a community. As it turns out, diffusion modeling evidence in recent years confirms these ideas: factors beyond individual differences can explain how far information travels and that network structure is important.

Watts[6] offered a spirited challenge to what he calls the "Influentials Hypothesis" by dispelling the idea that certain people are destined to be centrally important to information diffusion. In fact, he and a colleague[7,8] modeled simulations of the spread of information through a large network and looked at which assumptions about the role that a small number of individuals (or "influentials") play—relative to non-influentials—are vital to account for widespread information dispersion through the simulated systems they created. By and large, these researchers concluded that the exact properties of the small number of designated influentials did not matter as much as structural factors. Watts noted that "the reason is simply that when influence is propagated via some contagious process, the ultimate effects typically depend far more on the global structure of the network than on the properties of the individuals near the start" (p. 206). He further drew an analogy to forest fires, noting the importance of not simply an initial spark but also "a conspiracy of wind, temperature, low humidity, and combustible fuel that extends over large tracts of land" (p. 206).

We need to understand not only individual people as agents of social diffusion but also the environments in which those people live. At least two different aspects of environment or space are crucial. We can clearly describe a person's social network as an entity larger than that person as an individual, and describe it in terms of a collective entity. From this perspective, mathematical characteristics of a person's social network should affect the likelihood and type of interpersonal interaction that occurs in everyday life. On a somewhat different plane, the nature of predominant ideas in circulation proximal to a person's home, either in childhood or later in life, also should affect what is discussed. In other words, in a sense, cultural differences—

again larger than any individual person—should also forecast possibilities for conversation among dyads or groups rooted in a particular culture.

The Effects of Network Characteristics

The experiences of researcher Susan Morgan[9] with various interventions intended to encourage organ donation offers a worthy conundrum. Campaign staff explicitly designed many of the efforts she described to encourage family discussion about organ donation. After a number of years of doing that work, Morgan noted that workplace-based efforts tended to achieve the intended outcomes in terms of family discussion, whereas university-based efforts tended not to accomplish the intended outcomes. While there are numerous plausible explanations, one possibility involves the daily routines and subsequent conversational opportunities of the two categories of participants. Typically, people in a workplace environment not only interact with one another but also go home at the end of each workday to connect with people in their household. However, many college students often do not have that same daily interaction with family, especially not face-to-face interaction. So, simple lack of access to relevant others likely inhibits sharing information about organ donation, no matter how poignant the original message might be.

The impact of partner availability on whether conversation occurs—not just in terms of the presence of others but also in terms of the existence of functional relationships—becomes clear in light of some basic evidence. Sohn,[10] for example, presented useful evidence from the advertising and public relations arena. In short, he documented the impact of social network density on a person's reported intention to pass along information electronically to others in the network. In other words, whether a person intended to share advertised information depended on the extent to which their social network is dense with interconnections.

Similarly, Lee[11] looked at network density as part of a larger dissertation on public perception of organizations. This study assigned participants to a five-person group (or situational network, for the purpose of the study). Participants were then shown hypothetical stories regarding an energy company and given an opportunity to talk freely with others about the material. Lee's approach was clever because he asked beforehand for members of each group to rate the closeness of their existing relationships with other members in the group (using a graphing technique common in social network analysis). Some participants were strangers to one another and others were friends or acquaintances, so Lee was able to observe a range of different small networks (albeit constructed ones). Each small group varied in its density (or connectedness). In other words, some groups included people who all reported a relationship with one another, whereas others included no existing close relationships. Lee found, perhaps unexpectedly but importantly for our discussion, that participants in the relatively dense networks experienced richer and more intense conversation than participants in low-density networks. That is, no matter how excited a person may have been about the news stories she or he read, whether or not conversation flowed appeared to be at least partially a function of the presence of ready conversational partners.

The social diffusion literature offers at least one caveat when weighing the possibility that interconnections between *multiple* nodes in a network matter. In the late 1980s, Burt[12] published an elegant (and subsequently often-cited) paper that investigated mechanisms for social contagion with regard to medical innovations. Burt reanalyzed data from an earlier classic study on innovation adoption among medical professionals called *Medical Innovation*.[13] Burt demonstrated that while person-to-person contagion is a crucial pathway through which people become aware of and decide to adopt innovations, the spread of information through a network requires at least one connection point to an outside network. In fact, connection points leading into and out of a small network are more important to information flow overall than the existence of lots of connections between people within the small network. Consequently, in the case of simple information diffusion, the ties leading *into and out of* a small community matter more than if there are interconnections between all community members.

Might network structure also affect *what* is shared? Intriguing results by Sohn[10] suggested that is the case. In relatively less-dense networks, people in Sohn's study were less likely to intend to discuss critical or negative views with others about particular commercial products. In relatively dense networks, people were more likely to share negative information with others. This suggests that positively framed information may be more likely to travel among loosely affiliated people, whereas more interconnected groups will share and ruminate on negatively framed information. Sohn interpreted this pattern to suggest that the nature of a person's immediately salient network conditions their intention to share certain types of information. Criticism may travel more easily in interconnected circles because people think such information will be acceptable and deemed valuable, whereas the uncertainty posed by relatively disconnected networks may dampen a person's enthusiasm for spreading negative views or information that is considered to be negative.

Social Capital, Social Cohesion, and Available Community Ties

In considering how communities vary in their encouragement or discouragement of information sharing between people, we are quickly confronted with the concept of social capital. In brief, *social capital* entails the general notion that groups of individuals vary in the resources available to individuals in those groups as a function of social ties between group members. A pundit might suggest, for example, that success in developing greenway bicycle trails and sustainable neighborhood recycling centers could reflect underlying social capital because interconnectedness and trust in one another somehow matter for collective action to develop trails or build recycling centers. One might even reasonably argue that the term "social capital" has emerged as a potent meme or shorthand idea that has traveled far among pundits and commentators. The notion of social capital now appears in a wide range of social science research.[14-18]

A foundation for the discussion of social capital is Bourdieu's[19] original delineation of different forms of capital in which he distinguished between economic capital, typically considered in terms of monetary value, and social capital, which encompasses the actual or potential resources that stem from having a network of social relationships among members of a group. Being a member of a group means that one can share available resources and that there is a sort of capital to use or protect. Coleman[20,21] further conceptualized social capital as a community resource available to individuals in the *community* but not necessarily located in any one individual.

Despite the widespread adoption of the social capital concept (or perhaps in part because of it), researchers and pundits now often mention the idea of social capital in a cursory way without defining exactly what it means operationally. While such practice has allowed broad theoretical pronouncements—such as "social capital affects health outcomes"—empirical research on social capital has been hampered by conceptual ambiguity, partly because of a lack of appropriate macro-level data to measure the notion.[22] One of the problems that can arise from using an ambiguous phrase like "social capital" is that we lose sight of specific dimensions of communities and interactions between people that are glossed over by such a hazy, overarching, all-encompassing notion.

Recently, scholars have begun to identify and clarify different dimensions or aspects of social capital that are uniquely meaningful. We can make a distinction, for example, between what has been labeled bonding social capital versus bridging and linking social capital.[18,23] Bonding social capital typically refers to the presence or absence of ties within homogenous social networks, whereas bridging and linking social capital refers to the existence of cross-cutting ties between groups of people or between institutions that exist because of community organizations and organizational networks. In that distinction, we might see different opportunities for network-to-network diffusion, as bonding ties would appear to set up echo chambers, whereas bridging ties appear to offer more opportunity for information to pass from one group to another. Knowing that generic social capital is high in a community does not necessarily indicate potential for incoming and outgoing diffusion of information, as a completely insular enclave may nonetheless be viewed as high in social capital, vaguely defined.

Not all preexisting relationships between people are likely to be equally helpful as pathways for health and science information sharing. Nowhere is this clearer than in Curley's work on leveraging ties,[24] in which she distinguished between individuals in one's social circle who are a net drain versus those who can and do offer help and assistance. An uncle who offers little more than exposure to crime and depravity may need to be counted as a local tie but is not necessarily going to provide the type of uplifting information sharing sometimes connoted by the notion of social capital. As Portes[25] observed, network ties actually can limit communication with external groups and reinforce negative perceptions of those outside of the group. In light of these ideas, Curley argued that what scholars loosely call social capital only operates as a force for positive change or reinforcement insofar as a person's social network actually encourages reciprocal helping. That helping can come through relatively weak ties to people dissimilar to oneself or from people in one's more intimate and local circle; what matters is the availability of help.

For some critics, a general concept of social capital is simply not a worthwhile foundation for theory, in part because of the need for the types of caveats just outlined. Some scholars have argued that equation of social capital with warm-and-fuzzy feelings about where one lives or overall trust in one's neighbors wanders too far from the concept's roots as a description of inequality.[26,27] Bourdieu[19] originally emphasized the collective sum of nonmonetary *resources* in a group (which can vary dramatically between social and economic classes) as a marker of inequality rather than simply emphasizing the extent of reciprocal relationships among people. Carpiano[26] argued that we should turn away from broad notions of social capital to focus on the fundamental dimensions of what he calls social cohesion, including social ties, as antecedent to (but not the same as) broader social capital. Other researchers have followed that call to look at concrete and functional social ties, for example, by looking at social ties as a predictor of health outcomes.[28]

These conceptual debates are important because they help to remind us of the need to be specific in our theorizing and to justify particular factors when invoking them as explanations for peer-sharing differences. If our quest is to predict who will share health or science information with their peers, the essences of bonding, bridging, and linking social capital are all relevant. But ultimately, it is the overall structural availability of functional and preexisting ties that likely matters most. Bonds within a group should encourage sharing with other group members by any single group member who happens to be initially contacted by an external organization. Moreover, an atmosphere rich with connections between individuals and institutions could encourage individual faith and trust in local institutions and facilitate the introduction of people to others in their community who can interact fruitfully with that institution as well. Connection to a science museum mailing list across town may facilitate the spread of word about a free rain barrel construction event being held at the museum. At the same time, the more opportunities community members have to attend local social events (such as neighborhood block parties in many parts of the United States), the longer everyone's list will be of salient names of local people who may be eligible for information sharing.

So, what can we use as a community-level indicator for our multilevel model of information sharing? The amount of available community ties—the extent of preexisting, functional ties between members of a community—offers a relatively simple and coherent variable that plausibly is antecedent to, or a foundation of, the broader concepts of social cohesion or social capital.[29] Some communication researchers have begun to focus only on evident relationships or ties as a source of disparities,[30] but we also can look at network infrastructure, which leads us to a macro-level rather than individual-level explanation. Such an approach turns attention to structural *opportunities* for community member interaction rather than solely seeking the opinions of individuals about their neighbors.

Why Community Ties Should Affect Information Sharing

If we want to know why people designate other people for information receipt, we need to know the functions that information sharing could serve in highly connected contexts versus less well-connected contexts. Over and above the simple necessity of a tie between two people for intentional sharing behavior to occur, the availability of ties also should set the stage for sharing in a number of ways. At the very least, we can point to the environmental *salience of other people*, the *preponderance of volunteerism*, and local methods for choosing *leaders* as important considerations in determining which communities are most likely to demonstrate information sharing.

Living in a community in which people are aware of what other community members do and in which sharing with others is recognized as a positive act likely affects information diffusion from person to person. Perceptions of what one ought to do (sometimes called injunctive norms) appear to be most strongly predictive of behavior in situations in which a person thinks other people actually are paying attention to one's own behavior.[31] Moreover, as Beaudoin[23] argued, social norms (or perceptions of what behaviors others approve and perform themselves) are most cognitively salient among residents of communities that harbor relatively abundant community ties, as many ties offer numerous routine reminders of what others think. Consequently, in communities in which there are many preexisting ties to remind people of others' everyday existence and information needs, peer referral is perhaps simply more likely to be on people's minds as an option.

Volunteerism also is a force that should drive information sharing and referral. The act of sharing information with another person, absent any direct order or financial reward, is a volunteer act. Places with many ties between people likely witness lots of volunteer behavior. Communities rich in established connections between people likely attract and retain people who believe helping their neighbors is valuable not just as a way of adhering to injunctive norms but also because of perceived community benefit. A preponderance of altruistic tendency, in turn, should encourage the spread of any health and science information deemed to be helpful to community members. (Of course, not all information sharing is intended to be helpful, as people spread rumors to undermine rivals or to promote their own ideas.) Altruism (measured as perceived importance of helping others) is predictive of content sharing in various domains and should be in the present context as well. For example, altruism predicts forwarding content from online advertising campaigns and spreading advertising messages through word of mouth.[32,33]

Social identity scholars[34-36] have offered another explanation from the perspective of leadership motivation. When people are in contexts that constantly remind them of their group membership, they tend to endorse leaders who embody the beliefs and behaviors that define that group rather than leadership candidates who are not prototypical. Leaders who gain authority positions through such routes, in turn, have reason to continue to emphasize group membership and identification through their leadership actions. A leader of a highly interconnected community likely would find more value in trumpeting efforts to share beneficial information with many community members than would a leader whose followers have deferred out of apathy or who see little value in their neighbor's well-being.

Evidence of the utility of information sharing as currency for relationships resides in Brabham's study[37] of people's motivations for participation in crowdsourcing efforts to improve transit planning through public engagement. (By "crowdsourcing," Brabham and others mean simultaneously sending an invitation to a large number of people, usually via the Internet, to provide input on the assumption that a large net will capture more useful ideas than only enlisting one or two experts.) Brabham investigated why people would bother to post to an online application developed in support of the Next Stop Design project, a Federal Transit Administration program involving public understanding of engineering science that intended to solicit public input regarding transportation. This study found that people viewed such posting as an opportunity to be recognized by peers, to express oneself, and even to advance one's career by gaining recognition as an expert. Pure contribution for the sake of altruism, in other words, was not the only driving force for those who opted to participate in crowdsourcing.

What does all of this mean for communities that vary in available community ties? Social bonding and bridging opportunities likely remind community members of their group membership. Consequently, group membership generally should be more salient in places with more bonding and bridging opportunities. Moreover, community leaders in those settings should see value in regularly identifying and assisting group members. Referral or nomination of community members clearly offers one way to do that because the act literally involves both the identification of others in a group and an active provision of (at least potential) benefit to them. Therefore, we would expect sharing and referral behavior most often in places with many ties between people, where nomination of fellow community members can be currency for group leadership.

Community Endurance and Residential Stability

Oishi and colleagues,[38] building on earlier work by Kasarda and Janowitz,[39] recently proposed that socioecological factors should predict what they deemed "procommunity action." Working at the zip code level with US Census data, these researchers hypothesized that residential stability, measured as a function of the proportion of a zip code's population living in the same house for 5 or more years, should positively predict various procommunity actions, such as donating money to a state fund to protect natural resources or attending a local sporting event regardless of team performance. Overall, residential stability did predict procommunity behaviors, at least in part by increasing identification with one's community. Importantly, residential stability conceivably could act as a moderator of other community-level relationships.[40] Information sharing, for example, should be dependent on not only the present, day-to-day availability of community ties but also the sufficient endurance of such ties to permit knowledge of community members' history and contact information. Forwarding a text message, for example, requires knowing the intended target person's cell phone number.

Community Ties, Stability, and Peer Referral for Mammography: An Empirical Example

The strategy of viral marketing is a prime example to illustrate the constraining power of network size, scope, and connections. Several years ago, the Minnesota Department of Health developed the Refer a Friend program (discussed briefly already in Chapter 4) as a way to promote its free mammography service for uninsured and underinsured women. In general, the Refer a Friend program increased the number of women using the service and was an important alternative to simply advertising the effort on television or radio.

Success in reaching some new women with a peer-referral program, however, does not rule out the possibility that certain groups will demonstrate more referral than others. One aspect of potential disparity in the case of the Refer a Friend program in Minnesota involved both available community ties and residential stability. Specifically, we wondered whether differences between communities in the number of ties available within each community would affect the preponderance of peer referral. We also wondered whether the extent to which there is turnover in who lives in a community would affect referral. In other words, does it matter if people often move into and out of a neighborhood? Does the stability of a neighborhood affect people's likelihood of sharing information with others?

In a survey study of participants living across Minnesota, we studied neighborhoods (or zip codes, at least) in terms of how often women in an area nominated others to get mammography information when given the chance.[29] We predicted that nomination tendency for a particular zip code would be a function of available community ties and also expected the predictive power of available ties would be greatest in communities with relatively high residential stability (meaning lower turnover in home residence). We were able to measure residential stability using US census data available for individual zip codes. Capturing available community ties involved more decision-making and was a less straightforward task. We had to rely on secondary data and turned to data available through the National Center for Charitable Statistics on religious congregation density (regardless of specific religious affiliation), a strategy originally introduced by Derose.[18] Admittedly, religious congregations per capita are not a perfect indicator of the number of information-sharing pathways between people in a neighborhood. We proposed, nonetheless, that the greater the density of formal organization of people for community-building, the greater the likelihood of information sharing in that geographic area.

The study results supported the main hypotheses. Congregation density positively predicted nomination tendency both in bivariate analysis and in full regression models (using Tobit regression) and was most predictive in zip codes that were notably high in residential stability—that is, above the median. Based on the results, having a local infrastructure of social ties available in a community appears to be important in allowing the diffusion of available health care services in that community. In other words, the most internally well-connected communities are the ones most likely to freely share information among themselves about cancer screening opportunities when given the chance.

Relationship History

Besides individual differences, the nature of a relationship between two people or among a group of peers undoubtedly conditions the prospects for sharing information. Borgatti and Cross[41] proposed that the decision to seek advice or information from another person depends on what one has learned from past relationship history. Borgatti and Cross suggested that information seeking from another person is a function of knowledge of what the other person knows, the perceived value of that information, having timely access to that person, and the perceived cost of getting information from the person in question. The simple availability of others might not be sufficient, as it also may be the case that having a good existing relationship with the right people matters.

Certain conversations might be made easier by the existence of a long-standing relationship. A mother and daughter with a close relationship may find it easier to talk about birth control than more estranged family members would. At the same time, however, extensive relationship history between two people also can introduce ironic distance in the case of sharing information.

Everyday experience suggests that families vary in conversational permissiveness, as do small groups of friends and coworkers. Some of that variability involves past history. For example, traumatic incidents, long-standing grudges, power differentials, and the need for future harmony in daily interactions can all hamper the free flow of talk and information sharing that may otherwise occur. Knowing that a spouse is likely to erupt in anger over the suggestion to buy a new energy-efficient refrigerator because of recent financial worries certainly could make a conversation about energy much less likely than might occur between two people who know each other but who do not live together and depend on one another for daily interaction.

The innovative work of Emily Brennan[42] at the University of Melbourne is a good example. Brennan gathered a group of adults in the Australian state of Victoria and showed them anti-smoking advertisements as part of an experimental study. Importantly, she recruited pairs of people for the study and showed the advertisements to the pairs, who varied in the self-reported strength of their relationship. Brennan then videotaped the interaction between the two participants following exposure to an advertisement. She found that the reported closeness between the two participants mattered in terms of what exactly was discussed. Pairs who were relatively less-close friends were more likely than pairs who were close friends to discuss quitting smoking, which was the target action intended by the advertisements. Pairs who were close friends actually talked more about smoking. Brennan posited that, in part, the constraint of friendship explains this pattern. A close friend of a smoker is perhaps more likely to be aware of the sensitivity involved in discussing quitting than would be a more distant acquaintance. Moreover, a close friend may think there is more to lose in raising a sensitive topic than an acquaintance. Consequently, for difficult subjects, closeness in relationships may introduce distance from conversation initiation.

In general, the risk of conversational initiation—or of a decision to forward an e-mail or sign someone up to receive a flyer—may be greatest for people with the fewest friends and family to whom to turn. If an individual is not widely connected to myriad others but instead relies on a close few for comfort and engagement, it is conceivable that when that person sees provocative material on television or views such material online she or he will be relatively unlikely to rock the boat and start talking about it, especially if the message on television involves challenging group norms. Imagine the teenage girl who feels relatively isolated and reliant on just a handful of friends. No matter how inspired she may get about new information about dating violence she finds late at night on the Internet, this girl faces considerable risk in sharing that information with her small social circle unless she is certain it will be embraced. Information that challenges critically important links between people may find more difficult passage than information spreading through widespread networks in which any particular social link is not so vital in one's everyday social life.

Cultural Differences

The social network dynamics discussed throughout this book are prevalent around the globe and not simply in an American Facebook user's online profile. Researchers have noted, for instance, the importance of word-of-mouth referrals in promoting HIV testing in Kenya,[43] prescription drugs in New Zealand,[44] and disaster preparedness among linguistically isolated groups in the United States.[45] While much of our discussion is universal to humans around the world, it is important to acknowledge that cultural differences also present a community-level or environment-level factor that could foster disparities in interpersonal interaction and even in the role that such interaction plays in explaining decision-making and behavior.

Just as we all reside within particular social networks, we also each operate within at least one cultural context at any given point in time. Insofar as cultures are larger than an individual person, it is appropriate to suggest that culture represents an overarching, environmental dimension that might beckon constant talk about particular health and science topics for some people and that might dampen any interpersonal interaction on those same topics for others.

Fant,[46] writing about conversational norms in Scandinavian and Hispanic cultures, suggested that anyone having even basic familiarity with everyday talk in these cultural settings will note "spectacular differences" between the two. These differences lie not only in the basic rules of the game, as in turn-taking and other guidelines for interaction, but also in topical preferences and what tends to be foregrounded. Among the differences Fant observed are contrasts between the Hispanic cultural value of conversation as a bonding ritual in and of itself versus the Scandinavian cultural need for conversation to have a purpose in pursuit of a larger goal. He also noted the importance of indicating consensus and agreement in Scandinavian talk versus the allowance of disagreement as a standard possibility for any conversation in Hispanic talk. Fant is careful to present these differences in terms of tendencies rather than as absolute stereotypes, an important distinction given the potential for any discussion of culture to invite unduly simplified thinking. Regardless, the preponderance of such differences should have distinctly limiting effects on what is discussed typically in the different cultural settings.

From this perspective, Scandinavian conversation about technological innovation, such as household solar energy appliances, would seem limited to some extent to people focusing on the utility of the technology for a particular, clear, and obvious purpose. Recommendations as to what one should do may be limited only to recommendations that can help achieve a clear and immediate goal, such as finding a way to reduce a family's energy costs. Conversely, one might expect discussion involving social norms—the sense a person has of others judgment of their own behavior—to blossom more frequently in discussion in Hispanic settings, given the importance of conversation both as a social activity and as a venue where open disapproval is acceptable.

Culture itself is a concept ripe with ambiguity, both in definition and in accounts of its causal role in human behavior. For our purposes, think of culture as a network of ideas to which some people have repeated access as a result of geography or community membership. While that frame may not satisfy all culture scholars, it at least serves to designate the set of environmental influences that distinguish someone who grew up in Miami from someone who grew up in Oslo. Viewed from this perspective, the preponderance of key values, which are embedded in the norms of everyday interaction for two people within a particular culture, should forecast the likelihood of information to spread exponentially among people. The forecast is likely one of differences rooted at least in part in culture. Exactly how culture arises is a question outside the scope of this discussion. However, for our purposes, we can note that there are apparent differences in the ideas in circulation in various communities around the world and even within the same community at distinctly different points in time.

As one example, consider the notion of familism, a belief in the importance of family honor and familial interconnectedness prevalent, if not universal, in cultural contexts and settings ranging from Eastern European town squares[47] to Jordanian living rooms[48] to family gatherings among Mexican Americans.[49] People who grow up with a strong sense that family honor is at least as important as individual preferences may be more likely to face particular expectations about what is or is not appropriate for conversation. Insofar as sexuality among adolescent women outside of marriage is not condoned, practical conversations about birth control options or methods of protecting oneself against sexually transmitted diseases may be less commonplace. Innovations in maternal choice, such as the so-called morning-after pill, either may not be a topic of conversation in circles in which family honor is paramount or may be discussed primarily with regard to judgment about sexual behavior and family reputation.

We might expect, based on these examples, that strategic efforts to rely on peer referrals also will differ in effect as a function of cultural context. Schumann and collaborators[50] provided at least some support for this possibility by studying the perceived effectiveness of word-of-mouth referrals among students in eleven different contexts, including India, Thailand, Hong Kong, China, Australia, the United States, Mexico, Germany, the Netherlands, Poland, and Russia. While they found more commonality across cultures than hypothesized, they also found that word-of-mouth referrals appeared to have a stronger effect on customer evaluation in some contexts than in others. Specifically, word-of-mouth referrals mattered more in countries they classified as being higher in uncertainty avoidance.

Fortunately, we live in a world that affords opportunities for intercultural interaction. These confluences, however productive and often enjoyable, also undoubtedly sometimes invite something of a clash at the level of conversational norms. When the conversational partners include a physician and a patient, the gaps in expectations would seem to afford substantial miscommunication. Imagine a scenario in which an African-American female pharmacist in the suburbs of a major American city advises a recent elderly

Chinese male immigrant as to the side effects of a prescribed drug. Researchers have observed that many Chinese people are reluctant to discuss their personal health with people outside of their immediate family.[51] This poses a distinct hindrance for whatever conversation may be possible between the pharmacist and the patient, aside from any linguistic challenges. It is conceivable that the patient would avoid asking embarrassing questions or getting the clarification he needs as to how to use the drug. In this case, the meeting of two cultures, over and above the interaction of two people, might hinder conversation.

The Need for Contextual Understanding

As outlined in this chapter, there are multiple reasons why a person's location—in geographic space, in a social network, or in a particular cultural environment—can constrain or amplify that individual's opportunity to share ideas, thoughts, and logistical information with other people or to benefit from such sharing by others. Clearly, factors beyond an individual's personality or daily choices affect that individual's likelihood of being a network hub in the spread of information or even in the digestion of and discussion of information. Undoubtedly, people have some agency in locating themselves, for example, by moving to new neighborhoods or attempting to join new social circles. Moreover, people can and do seek information on their own through Internet searches and trips to the library. However, this sense of mobility and possibilities for information seeking does not eradicate the real differences between community contexts that appear to exist with regard to information sharing. These discrepancies, in turn, appear to be subtle factors that help to shape the information populating a person's everyday life. With a person's situation and context in mind, we now can turn to factors related to *content* and how those may affect what is shared and what is not.

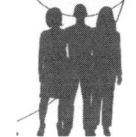

CHAPTER 6

What Information Matters: Content-Level Factors That Affect Sharing

In addition to our exploration of individual-level and community-level factors that constrain information sharing, we can examine yet another level of analysis by again using the example of why talk about scientific research related to Hurricane Sandy was not universal or even necessarily widespread among the US population in fall 2012. Previous chapters looked at various ways individual characteristics predispose people to be more or less likely to share information with others and discussed community-level differences. This chapter will focus on variables that describe messages themselves.

Some aspects of the Hurricane Sandy story and others like it may invite peer-to-peer sharing more than others. Consider the temptation to forward photographs of the damaged New Jersey shoreline to friends who you know have visited there before versus the disinclination many may have to forward a lengthy scientific paper on the effects of ocean temperature. Moreover, as I noted earlier, entertainment stories such as the sale of the *Star Wars* franchise appear to have been roughly as popular as Hurricane Sandy across the United States as fodder for Twitter during the days after the storm made landfall. This suggests that even the general topic of Hurricane Sandy may not have been the most popular topic in some discussion circles. Perhaps for many people, Yoda trumps climate science as a cue for conversation.

Consequently, this chapter will assess what we know about *message factors* that prompt or discourage sharing and discussion. Many health and science stories may be hindered in their ability to ignite information spread in viral fashion by their topic or by the way they are presented and framed.

Any thorough consideration of people's routine conversations and sharing must at some point confront the fact that people do not talk about every topic equally as often. Certain topics tend to animate our everyday interactions with others more than other topics. Colleagues and I found this pattern, for example, in trying to understand parent interactions with teenagers regarding indoor tanning.[1] After recruiting people to talk about their typical tanning conversations, it became apparent that many mothers and daughters do not spend a lot of time discussing the scientific literature on the health effects of tanning. Instead, insofar as there was any relevant discussion at all, most interaction tended to focus on the logistics of where to find a tanning salon, coupons or sale offers, the financial expense of tanning, or other relatively mundane, but practically oriented, ideas. When it comes to sharing information with friends and family, certain messages appear to be more predictable as candidates to travel farther than others.

Two examples, pulled at random from the daily stream of news features that various news outlets now regularly post as part of the ephemeral torrent of bits and bytes online, hint at our information sharing habits. The *Washington Post* regularly posts the top 20 most e-mailed news stories among its national audience. On a more local level, the *News & Observer* (based in Raleigh, North Carolina) offers a similar list of the most e-mailed stories as well as the most read (at least as measured by Internet views). This tracking of e-mailed stories is regular practice now for numerous news outlets. The lists are sufficiently ubiquitous that we might take them for granted as useful sources of information, even if we glance at them as a guide to popular news. A deeper look, however, is revealing.

A list of the most e-mailed stories in the *Washington Post* on a day in summer 2012 appears in Table 1. The list includes a wide variety of topics. Health or science stories certainly are not predominant on the list. Health-related or science news stories that do appear tend to be of a particular type. For instance, there is a story regarding—in an intriguingly reflexive turn given the focus of this book—the viral spread of a judge's supposed missive regarding health care and a story on Singapore's health care system. There is also a story on poison ivy treatment, one on the link between stress and aging, and several offering recommendations for concentration improvement and ways to live a better life. The majority of these stories focus on tips for the everyday health of readers. Those that do not offer tips are linked to the national debate over health care reform that animated news coverage in the United States in the wake of the Supreme Court decision regarding the Affordable Care Act mentioned in Chapter 1. This example of what is forwarded—albeit a single example—suggests three initial ideas about information sharing: (1) much information sharing regarding news stories does not involve health or science information; (2) much of the information sharing involving medical research or other scientific research that does occur focuses on personal health tips and recommendations that stem from such research; and (3) controversies and ongoing debates in the news, such as those surrounding health care, will stir up information sharing among at least some corners of regular news readers. What is less apparent from this list is what is *not* listed. For example, stories about topics on which there is tremendous scientific consensus or stories not squarely focused on individual (rather than collective) well-being are absent, among other items.

Table 1. Stories e-mailed the most in the *Washington Post* on July 30, 2012

1. "A judge's letter on health care and an email gone viral"
2. "Down in the Weeds"
3. "The Register Endorsement: How Clinton Won It and What It Means"
4. "Our GIs Earn Enough"
5. "Quranic Values as an Inspiration for Gay Marriage"
6. "Europeans Investigate CIA Role in Abductions"
7. "Choose Your Poison Ivy Treatment"
8. "Singapore's Model"
9. "Carolyn Hax Live: Advice columnist tackles your problems"
10. "The Fix Live"
11. "Want to get that house off your hands as quickly as possible? Here's how"
12. "The gift of the Gores"
13. "Top Secret America"
14. " Spice: Sriracha"
15. "Question 3: Do colleges want well-rounded students or those with a passion?"
16. "Ginnifer Goodwin is Snow White"
17. "Doodle? Do, to Improve Concentration"
18. "Who Is"
19. "12 Ways to Live a Better Life"
20. "Study is First to Confirm That Stress Speeds Aging"

Source: www.washingtonpost.com, accessed July 30, 2012. Capitalization and story headlines are as they appeared.

Next, looking at the stories that were read the most and e-mailed the most in the *News & Observer* on the same summer day, the focus for the North Carolina paper was understandably somewhat more local than the *Washington Post*. Regardless, certain patterns again are clear, and we can see some distinctions between what people read and what they choose to forward to other people they know via e-mail. Table 2 lists the stories that were read the most and e-mailed the most on that given day.

Table 2. Stories read the most and e-mailed the most in the *News & Observer* (Raleigh, North Carolina) on July 30, 2012

Stories most read	Stories most e-mailed
1. "State government salaries"	1. "Wilber's marks 50 years of barbecue"
2. "Loaded field to swim 'Race of Century'"	2. "Closed to public, Orton Plantation is transforming on a 'grand scale'"
3. "Former Wake judge pleads guilty on altered DWI cases"	3. "UNC-Chapel Hill faculty calls for outside review of athletics and academics"
4. "University employee salaries"	4. "Report: UNC-Chapel Hill athletic advisers steered players to classes"
5. "Citrix's move downtown could transform Raleigh's warehouse district"	5. "Upscale restaurants bloom in Eastern N.C."

Source: www.newsobserver.com, accessed July 30, 2012. Capitalization and story headlines are as they appeared.

Comparing these two lists reveals that the stories that the most people read were not at all the same as the stories that the most people e-mailed to others. Again, this example offers a single snapshot of a local media market. Nonetheless, it is useful to note that news stories that draw people's reading attention do not necessarily produce forwarding and information sharing.

Beyond that, we might start to characterize the types of stories on the two lists. Generally, many of the stories on the most read lists involve surveillance in some way, whether prurient monitoring of others' salaries or environmental scanning of recent crimes and business developments. Stories on the most e-mailed lists, however, tend to focus on socialization and judgment. Many of the most e-mailed stories appear to involve social bonding opportunities focused on local places of entertainment that may serve as prompts for discussion with family or friends about what to do on the upcoming weekend. Other stories involve recent controversies in the news, such as lapses in judgment by the athletic department at an elite university.

Surveillance, socialization, and discussion of controversy all fit Charles Wright's decades-old framework[2] describing the various functions that mass media news coverage serves for societies. Much of the peer-to-peer information sharing, nonetheless, appears to involve what is directly pertinent to the social aspects of everyday life or to ongoing debates or discussions one might have with friends. News stories that do not involve either a direct threat to individual or family well-being or opportunity for social interaction seem less likely to spread via e-mail and online forwarding, at least in this example.

Nuanced judgments aside about exactly which stories are most likely to be forwarded, at least one overarching idea is clear from these initial examples. Not all news stories are created equal in their potential to be shared. From that conclusion, we can speculate that messages are not all equally likely to be discussed, reposted on Facebook, or retweeted via Twitter. Some empirical research and theory development helps to explain why this may not be the case. For instance, certain topics seem to invite greater tendency toward disparity in dispersion and commentary than others. Himelboim[3] found that health-related online discussion boards demonstrated more unequal distribution of responses across initial posts than political discussions. A small number of health posts tended to attract much of the total commentary in this study, whereas political posts were more evenly distributed in posted responses. Himelboim speculated that people searching for facts related to a disease may scan threads but then just look at the most popular posts, assuming those to be most credible, and only add comments there. Political commentators, however, may be more willing to engage a range of postings for the sake of entertainment and general advocacy.

Importantly, the notion that some material may simply be more likely, on average, to be shared stands somewhat in contrast to the notion that *individual*-level characteristics drive information sharing. Such an idea resonates with critics who have argued against the idea that only certain kinds of people are vital in understanding information diffusion.[4] At the same time, even within a theoretical exploration of message factors are the roots of an argument for disparities between people.

Morgan,[5] drawing on the social representations literature,[6] suggested that for an idea to leap from the television screen into everyday discourse there needs to be some degree of integration of what is broadcast with existing daily discourse among people. This means that, in part, a message must be more than dry exposition of a fact and somehow resonate with the narratives that populate our lives as dreaming and yearning human beings. We tend to engage information that is shaped into a story more readily and hungrily, for instance, than the pages and pages of useful but not sequentially compelling information in a printed phone book.

Some commentators actually privilege ideas over people as powerful agents of propagation. Earlier, we encountered the notion of the meme as a replicable idea that can operate in some ways like a gene. Blackmore[7] went so far as to argue that human beings are essentially meme machines, whereby people in this formulation serve to carry forward memes rather than vice versa. Even

such perspectives, however, recognize the importance of understanding
the unique nature of human hosts in the process of propagation. Dawkins[8]
suggested that the success of a meme should be a function of its appeal to,
or resonance with, the structure of human brains as well as the ease of its
replication. Blackmore deftly considered the very idea of a "meme" as a meme
itself, suggesting that its own longevity over time may be because of the
similarity between the four-letter word *meme* and the already well-established
concept of a *gene*. Resonance with existing human knowledge, as well as the
ability to leverage human tendencies, seems to be vital.

At least two aspects of human tendency are relevant in theorizing about
successful meme diffusion: human response to open-ended information
presentation and the impact of emotion. We can see the value of considering
the former by thinking about what rhetoric scholars have observed for
centuries since Aristotle. The importance of the latter will be apparent in
describing the role of arousal in prompting human interaction. Beyond those
two dimensions, we also can look at the value of messages that generally boost
confidence and self-esteem, especially with regard to understanding scientific
research.

Does Rhetorical Structure Matter?

One factor to consider that can invite or discourage subsequent interpersonal
interaction is the very structure or form of information. A theoretical essay
by Hoeken and colleagues[9] on the role of what they called the influence
of rhetorical tropes can shed some light on this. They suggested that a
particular message form can prompt subsequent conversation. Whether a
message functions to entice people to talk about the ideas in question is likely
constrained in some way by its form. Importantly, these constraints also
suggest that certain people are more predisposed to talk about specific health
and science material in certain ways, which I will explain.

Hoeken and colleagues focused on the experience of an HIV testing
campaign in South Africa run by an organization called loveLife. Campaign
messages directly address the social nature of sexual behavior and invite the
audience to think about social interaction. Hoeken and co-authors argued that
the formal manner in which the campaign materials addressed the audience
made interpersonal interaction more likely.

Central to this argument is the notion of a rhetorical ellipsis, or a truncated
premise that leaves at least part of its intended meaning implicit rather than
explicitly stated. Two example phrases from the campaign[9] are "No until

we know" (or "NO 'til we know") and "If it's not just me, you're not for me." Implicit in the first message is the idea that one should refuse sexual encounters with a partner until that partner's HIV status is known. Implicit in the second message is the idea that if a sex partner is not being monogamous that she or he is not suitable as a partner. Gleaning the intended meaning is not guaranteed in either case, as the audience member would need to do some work interpreting and understanding the message, especially relative to simpler messages such as "Only have sex with HIV-tested people" or "Don't tolerate sexual polygamy."

The rhetorical value of the truncated premise is an idea dating back at least to Aristotle[10] who, like his fellow students of rhetoric, believed that implying part of your argument and requiring the audience to fill in the blank was more persuasive than complete statement of all premises in an argument. Consider a three-part claim that humans are changing the climate, that climate change will threaten human existence, and therefore humans should do something to reverse or mitigate the danger. Now consider the two-part claim that humans are changing the climate and humans should do something to reverse or mitigate the danger. Aristotle, while likely agnostic as to climate change prospects in his day, would likely argue that the latter formulation has the advantage of inviting the audience to assume a harm without having to spell it out, thereby inviting the audience to fill in the blank with ideas about potential consequences. Similarly, the argument by Hoeken and colleagues about the value of the ellipsis depends on audiences' filling in the blank and thereby participating in message interpretation more than they otherwise would.

Being able to identify a meaningful interpretation for such messages likely prompts self-congratulatory thoughts among audience members.[9,11,12] That boost of self-confidence and understanding, in turn, can encourage conversations that serve as an outlet through which to share this newly discovered meaning and demonstrate one's knowledge to others. In some ways, the argument harkens back to my previously mentioned work with Torres on the importance of perceived topical understanding in encouraging talk.[13]

At the same time, in offering these insights about message structure, Hoeken and colleagues also offered the seeds of an argument for likely disparity by discussing anecdotal evidence from the loveLife experience that suggests some people shied away from talking about campaign materials they did not understand. Individuals who did not get the intended implicit reference were actually less likely, in those instances, to chat with others about the messages or the key ideas. In other words, the same message structure that can be viewed as soliciting talk and information sharing among some individuals may also dissuade others from conversing or sharing with others.

Is There a Role for Emotional Response?

The literature on evaluation of public health promotion campaigns around the world yields a different idea about a type of message that may invite conversation. Specifically, evidence suggests that especially provocative or sensational images can prompt sharing with others. In Australia, for example, exposure to graphic imagery in anti-smoking advertisements has predicted tendency to talk about those advertisements.[14] In a different example from Norway, an anti-smoking campaign used provocative, emotional appeals to stimulate conversation among adolescent viewers and their peers.[15] In approaching the audience, campaign planners assumed that people (and more specifically adolescents) tend to tell their friends, family, and neighbors about particularly startling media content that they encounter. They likely do so, in part, because of their need for interpersonal bonding in moments of vulnerability or excitement.

What drives conversation in response to provocative content? Dunlop, Kashima, and Wakefield[16] studied friendship dyads (pairs of friends) in Australia who saw advertisements promoting a vaccination for the human papillomavirus, or HPV. They then tracked the extent to which participants talked, both immediately and for a period following the viewing. Participants either saw a relatively straightforward, or expository, public service announcement that stated reasons for seeking HPV vaccination, or they saw an advertisement that used a narrative format that relied to a greater extent on storytelling. The findings did not show that general advertisement format mattered in predicting the likelihood of subsequent conversation. Participants who saw the narrative advertisement and those who saw the expository advertisement were comparable in their tendency to talk with others about the topic. What the study did find, however, was that participants' *emotional* response—the extent to which they reported fear, anxiety, or worry—did predict their likelihood of talking with others following the advertisement exposure.

Emotional response appears to prompt people to turn to friends or family, perhaps for comfort, information seeking, or normative assessment. Brennan[17] replicated this finding, for example, in her work on anti-smoking advertisement response in Australia. This study found that emotional response to anti-smoking advertisements positively predicted tendency to talk about the advertisements. Over and above reasoning as to the logic of arguments presented in media content, the extent to which one's heartstrings are tugged or passion is inflamed appears to matter in predicting who will turn to their peers after reading or viewing or hearing information.

Work by Berger and colleagues at the University of Pennsylvania went even further to establish the apparent role of emotion in information sharing. Berger provided evidence that people who are more physiologically aroused will be more likely to share information with others, in part because their excited state mobilizes neural resources involved in sharing and interpersonal engagement. In two separate studies, Berger[18] found that people who have watched emotion-engaging videos are more likely to share information with others afterward, as are people who jog. Both video watching and jogging boosted general arousal, which in turn appears to have increased people's reported willingness to share information with friends, family members, and coworkers.

Berger and Milkman[19] analyzed a large number of articles from *The New York Times* that appeared on the most e-mailed lists, a large-scale version of the single example analyses from the opening of this chapter. (See also Schriner[20] for another look at most-e-mailed news stories.) Berger and Milkman coded stories by the extent to which the material was emotionally charged. Essentially, the findings indicated that content that evokes "high-arousal emotions"—such as awe, anger, or anxiety—is more likely to spread virally than content that largely invites low arousal, which is likely to invite sadness, for example. Berger and Milkman concluded that low-arousal content is less likely to inspire direct action than high-arousal content.

Provoking emotional response, however, is far from a panacea for unfettered information spreading. Inviting emotion, particularly emotion with a negative valence, can invite unintended consequences. Human beings tend to engage one another in response to emotion. A number of social psychologists have found greater tendency toward conversation when people are coping with certain emotions.[21,22] This pattern of reaching out to others in moments of confusion or alarm is consistent with the long history of studies on rumors and gossip that can be traced back at least to Allport and Postman's post–World War II book *The Psychology of Rumor*.[23] More recently, colleagues and I assessed the uptick in information seeking that followed news coverage of the controversy and confusion surrounding mammography guidelines in 2009.[24] Much of the discussion we seek with others in moments of elevated emotion, however, is not necessarily focused on new factual information sharing as much as it is focused on reassurance, coping with stress, and ritualistic bonding.

The role of emotion in information sharing also is complicated by the scholarly realization that emotional response not only varies in terms of sheer arousal but also, potentially, in terms of qualitative experience. Many emotion theorists posit that we can experience a range of what might be called discrete emotions.[25,26] In other words, many have argued that we do not simply feel positively or negatively, but we are capable of a range of subtly different emotional states, such as anger, happiness, sadness, or even surprise. These discrete states likely are rooted in evolution[26]; we have emotion, at least in part, to prompt response to threats and opportunities in our environment. An anger response may be adaptive in enabling us to fight back against an attacking animal. Happiness can encourage relaxation and a steady state. Different emotional responses seem to invite different action tendencies.

This suggests that different emotional responses will not equally produce conversation initiation. Some states will be more likely to lead to sharing with friends or family than other states. In fact, Peters, Kashima, and Clark[27] recently found precisely that pattern with their study of story sharing. People were more likely to engage others when disgusted, surprised, or happy relative to moments, for example, when they were sad or contemptuous.

These human tendencies are noteworthy in the case of advertising campaigns intended to spark supportive conversations about eating healthily or recycling or other behaviors. If we accept that people often talk to one another as a method of defending their own ego, soothing hurt feelings, or calming their nerves, then we also can expect at least some interpersonal interaction that will undermine the intentions of message designers and campaign planners. (Chapter 7 further explores this possibility.)

Can Messages Boost Confidence in Talking With Others?

Another reason certain messages might lead to interpersonal conversation is that exposure to messages may boost a person's sense of topical understanding and conversational competency. If a message raises people's confidence (rightly or not) in their ability to understand and talk about a particular topic, then, all other factors being equal, we can expect that talk about that topic will be more likely to ensue. It may be the case that certain message presentations are simply better than others at instilling confidence in understanding among the audience. At least one of the studies discussed earlier sheds empirical light on this question.

As part of the previously mentioned science television news multiyear project described in Chapter 4, Alicia Torres of the American Institute of Physics and I surveyed a television news audience to determine the impact of seeing news stories that had been specially crafted to boost their personal sense of understanding of science and math. The findings suggested not only that short television news stories, presented as part of a typical local television news program, could increase viewers' sense of understanding but also that such confidence was important in predicting who among the audience subsequently would turn to family and friends to discuss various science topics. In general, could well-crafted news stories get people talking, or would the same people who usually talk just continue to do so?

Evidence from experimental results discussed earlier and subsequent data from a national survey indicated that the nature of media content can affect subsequent conversation about the topic at hand.[11,28] To understand why, it is useful to understand something about the project we evaluated, known as *Discoveries and Breakthroughs Inside Science* (DBIS). The project, run by the American Institute of Physics, received support from the National Science Foundation to produce a syndicated science news service available to local television stations in a number of markets around the United States. DBIS offers a broad spectrum of research news by working with a coalition of science, technology, engineering, and mathematics organizations, including universities and research institutions. Coalition organizations help produce peer-reviewed, multidisciplinary television news reports, offering an outside review standard not typically witnessed in most newsrooms. Typical DBIS stories in this study can be categorized into three major areas: earth and atmospheric sciences, medical advances, and physical sciences and engineering. Stories were distributed monthly to television stations across the country for use in local programming. Perhaps most importantly, DBIS reporters attempted to explain recent scientific research in plain language and to emphasize the connection between scientific results and everyday life in the United States.

When interpreting the results described in Chapter 4, it is crucial to remember that the specific news stories in question had been designed to make scientific research accessible and to be relevant to television news viewers' everyday lives. Not all television news content necessarily strives to boost confidence in that fashion (though much of it is crafted with an eye toward audience expectations for relevance). Nonetheless, there is evidence here that certain kinds of educational content, all other factors being equal, may generally encourage discussion. Such evidence suggests at least some promise for widespread sparking of conversation. At the same time, it is important to note that the effect sizes observed in this study were not especially large. Even with regard to specially crafted science news stories, many people did not discuss the programming or relevant topics at all.

Incentive Offers for Peer Referral

Advertising messages and other presentations of information sometimes include an explicit invitation to share the news with friends or family members. Some viral marketing efforts even take the invitation a step further by offering an incentive to people to entice them to spread the word. In the context of health- or science-related information, explicit incentives—such as an offer of money in exchange for the contact information of friends or family members— may encourage more peer referral than otherwise might occur. But we need to know more about the quality and nature of that referral.

Several colleagues and I looked precisely at the issue of financial incentives to increase peer referral as a part of the larger set of efforts described earlier to promote mammography. Specifically, we wondered whether *paying* people for the names and contact information of relevant others in their social network would help to accomplish program goals. We found that the question of incentive utility may ultimately need to be judged as a function of what exactly are the program goals. Paying people appears to yield somewhat different results than relying on people's willingness to volunteer.

We designed an experiment that compared the impact of incentives on peer nomination among people who previously had participated in a mammography program. Women were offered a $20 incentive each time someone they referred to the program was screened, a $5 incentive for each name and valid address or phone number submitted (regardless of screening completion), or no financial incentive for nomination.[29] Offering $5 per nomination yielded the most nominations per referral invitation sent, compared with the $20 per completed mammogram group and the no incentive group. In the no incentive condition, however, each participant who made referrals generated as many or more scheduled mammograms on average as did participants in the $20 per completed mammogram group or the $5 per name group. The results suggested that the nature of the peer referral that occurs when people are paid differs from that which happens when people simply decide to volunteer to refer the material. The extent to which financial incentives are presented or offered may affect the referral behavior that is actually prompted. This is yet another way in which message framing and content also are relevant to our discussion.

The Case for Message-Level Differences

This chapter entertained the idea that certain types of materials are more likely to be shared, or at least to prompt conversation. Evidence suggests differences between content that is more versus less elliptical, more versus less emotionally provocative, or more versus less confidence-boosting. Even in an analysis of differences between messages in their ability to prompt interpersonal interaction, however, we can find the roots of an argument for our tendency toward disparity absent planning or intervention. Material that relies on implicit premises will be more easily interpreted, and thus acted upon by some people, for example. Certain information, at least certain message presentations, may be more likely to travel than other general information. In noting that all content does not seem equally likely to prompt sharing, we also are left with yet more evidence that people are not likely to be equal vessels, as whether you share seems to partly depend on that information to which you happen to encounter in everyday life.

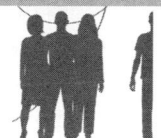

CHAPTER 7

The Consequences of Information Sharing

What are the consequences of the various information-sharing patterns explored in this book? Do the gaps in information-sharing tendencies between individuals, groups, and communities represent problems to be addressed or are they simply observable reflections of our clustered and networked world? Based on what we examined in Chapters 4 through 6, we have a host of reasons to expect that information somehow released into the world will not spark a uniform chorus of peer-to-peer dispersion. A key question is whether that heterogeneity is of consequence.

To appreciate the ways in which information-sharing differences are consequential, it is useful to think about systems and networks and not simply about individuals. People can serve as inputs for those around them. Especially in the absence of prevalent mass media coverage of issues, who it is that you know (and how able and likely they are to share information with you) can directly affect the information environment in which you live and operate on a daily basis. In turn, the extent to which information reaches your neighbors and stops there is noteworthy.

A hypothetical example serves to illustrate these considerations. Imagine two adults, Dawn and Shawn, each in their forties and living in average-sized metropolitan areas on opposite coasts of the United States. One day, each of them walks into a local hardware store and picks up a pamphlet touting the benefits of LED (light-emitting diode) light bulbs as a replacement for conventional incandescent light bulbs. Within 3 months, 75 people that Dawn knows have adopted LEDs in their homes, whereas no one Shawn knows (other than himself) has done so. Contemplating what may have happened provides a chance to review a set of possibilities explored in this book.

Assume for the moment that there was no mass media campaign promoting LED bulbs in either Dawn or Shawn's area. Also assume that the pamphlet was the most prominent piece of material in either area. Further, assume that Dawn and Shawn are the only people in their respective networks who happened to see the pamphlet promoting LED bulbs. Additionally, we can productively speculate by ignoring the possibility that people in Shawn's network are somehow heavily invested in the incandescent bulb industry or otherwise predisposed against LED bulbs. What if the differences in adoption of the use of LED bulbs lie in discrepancies in information sharing initiated (or not) by Dawn and Shawn?

Perhaps Dawn is more outgoing than Shawn. Perhaps the pamphlet found a willing champion when Dawn happened upon it. If that was the end of the story, we would have reason to caution viral marketing professionals, but relatively little cause for some of the concerns raised in previous chapters. We may worry more, however, about differences attributable to the local environments in which Dawn and Shawn each grew up and in the nature of their existing networks. Imagine that Dawn and Shawn are equally comfortable talking to other people in general and equally excited by the new LED bulb. What if the difference in engagement with others about the bulb stemmed from the paucity of people in Shawn's network? What if Shawn was not as comfortable bringing up the issue of light bulbs among friends because his primary interaction with friends happens in settings such as Saturday afternoon football viewing that do not typically invite such discussion? On a different plane, what if Dawn felt more comfortable explaining how the LED bulb works?

If widespread adoption of LED technology is a goal, and if government mandate is not a ready option, disparity in peer-to-peer interaction between Dawn's network and Shawn's network is consequential. Keep in mind that it is *the people close to Dawn and Shawn*, not simply Dawn or Shawn, who will demonstrate many of the effects of information-sharing disparities. If Shawn is not active in talking with others about the LED bulb innovation, we need to look for the impact of that inactivity on the consequent information salience for other people around him. Low adoption by Shawn's network in the aggregate would likely persist no matter how successful the pamphlet may be in affecting Shawn's own behavior in his own living room. Ultimately, we can see at least some evidence of impact in the contrast between the LED bulbs populating the houses of Dawn's contacts and the lack of use of such bulbs in houses of people who know Shawn.

Exactly how innovation adoption patterns come to pass as a result of peer-to-peer interaction likely involves more than direct persuasion by Dawn or Shawn of their neighbors and families. Structural, educational, or situational information-sharing differences may have produced the stark innovation adoption differences between Dawn's circle of connections and Shawn's circles of connections in a variety of other ways as well. This chapter outlines some of those differences.

Setting aside (until Chapter 8) whether we should intervene to address disparities, we should ask why and how the information-sharing disparities could have noteworthy effects. Why should we care if any two people are drastically different in either their tendency to share with others or their exposure to peer referrals? Several distinct outcomes serve to answer these challenges. On a basic level, we need to address the possibilities for differential growth in knowledge between various groups over time. The consequences of interpersonal interaction for subsequent audience knowledge and behavior are not limited to issues of knowledge acquisition, as a wide array of possibilities are plausible.[1]

Knowledge Gain

One outcome of consequence for the types of disparities in interpersonal interaction noted throughout this book is a straightforward one. Variation in the amount and type of interpersonal interactions to which a person has access ought to affect that person's access to knowledge. On a basic level, we can point back to our earlier discussion of the knowledge gap hypothesis.[2] In general, individuals with more prior information exposure (whether from newspapers, textbooks, or knowledgeable colleagues) ought to outstrip those who do not enjoy such resources in additional knowledge gain over time.

Public health campaigns offer one context in which it appears that connections between people matter as a conduit of exposure. Using data from a study conducted in the Netherlands, van den Putte and colleagues[3] demonstrated that talk between people can serve as a bridge whereby those who were not directly exposed to an original broadcast message nevertheless can hear about the broadcast information from someone who was exposed. Researchers surveyed Dutch smokers over time and found that a mass media campaign prompted interpersonal conversation that subsequently was associated with intention to quit smoking and quit attempts even among smokers who *were not directly exposed* to the original campaign. In other words, the campaign had an indirect effect on ideas about smoking cessation by virtue of prompting conversations.

At the same time, we can make a more subtle argument for the impact of routine network interactions on knowledge gain over time. William "Chip" Eveland's investigation of what he called anticipatory elaboration is noteworthy here. The short story is that the preparation you do in getting ready to go home for Thanksgiving—quickly scanning the latest sports news to be able to talk with your niece, who is a diehard women's soccer fan—can be a noteworthy prompt for information gain beyond the actual learning that may occur during the dinner-table talk that unfolds.

Eveland's research cautions us against assuming that social networks lead to unfettered diffusion of information through talk alone. Much of Eveland's work focused on politics and civic life in the United States. Among other puzzles, he has sought to understand how exactly interpersonal communication might be so consistently related to key variables such as knowledge[4,5] without it necessarily being the case that talk is simply a link through which new information flows from the knowledgeable to their followers. At least three plausible explanations could account for the often-documented relationship between knowledge about politics and talk about politics: simple exposure (or a diffusion account in which knowledge spreads from those in the know to others), anticipatory elaboration, and discussion-generated elaboration.

According to Eveland, a simple exposure explanation would mean that talking with a person exposes others to information to which that person previously has been exposed; that is, one person passes information to the next. Elaboration explanations offer somewhat different accounts. In a situation of anticipatory elaboration, people are motivated to process information they encounter (or seek) more deeply when they anticipate impending conversations with others. Eveland also argued for the possibility of discussion-generated elaboration, an idea that focuses on information processing at the actual time of the conversation in question.

In one study, Eveland[6] used US election survey data and found the most support for elaboration explanations. People appeared to prepare for talk by elaborating on information beforehand. Mere anticipation of future conversations, as well as actual discussion with others, apparently can prompt information seeking and learning. However, Eveland did not find as much support for the simple exposure account. While he discovered a positive relationship between political discussion and political knowledge, he did not identify any additional boost in knowledge from speaking with a relatively knowledgeable partner. Eveland's work does not rule out the possibility of diffusion (or the two-step flow) altogether, but it does suggest that in some domains, like politics, in which debate is anticipated, living in certain networks can inspire people to learn simply so that they come to the table prepared. Conversely, individuals who do not anticipate any such challenges may have less motivation to gain information. Sometimes, anticipated interaction prompts media use and information seeking rather than just acting as a source of new information.

Cognitive Salience

We know that human memory, for better or worse, is not a perfect reflection of an objective reality through which somehow we pass and collect thoughts to be stored. Our processing, storage, and retrieval of experience is richer and more complex than that. Among the filters that affect our relationship to the past are the daily interactions we have with one another in the present.

Everyday conversation is related to our basic memory for various events.[7-9] People do not always store information directly from their lives and then simply retrieve that information later in unmitigated fashion. For example, a late-night conversation on one's cell phone or an animated discussion at the dinner table or an exchange via an online chat application may affect how people remember what came before that talk.

How is it that a mundane exchange with a lover or a coworker or a distant relative matters to our mental images of the past? Memory comprises a complex of subsystems that are vulnerable to a variety of influences.[10] We can understand memory as an umbrella notion that encompasses processes such as encoding (or recording) and later retrieval, and *retrieval* is one aspect of memory on which conversation can have a distinct effect.

When we remember an idea, a name, or a face, we are activating information that otherwise is lying quietly in our brains. To our consternation (or salvation), retrieving a memory almost never results in a perfectly efficient procurement of a single representation. Instead, the stimulus that prompted retrieval, such as phrase or a question in a conversation with another person, invites remembering an array of related thoughts. As Fuster[11] succinctly noted, "that stimulus, in a broad sense, is like the hand in the basket that picks out one cherry and makes others follow"(p. 199).

That lovely metaphor enjoys a host of empirical support. Anderson's pioneering work to describe network models of memory painted a picture of remembering in which we access information in our brain through activation of interconnected neural nodes.[12,13] Again, networks return to our discussion, this time residing in our gray matter rather than among our Facebook pages. Our brain architecture allows for spillover activation of adjacent nodes whenever a node is activated. Wirtz[14] explored this possibility and found that simply talking with another person can temporarily activate a mindset, such as one's sense of identity as an athlete or as a student, that subsequently influences one's later evaluation of media messages. Activation of one specific node also will enhance the salience of related information in adjacent nodes, which is part of the basis for expecting memory enhancement. Moreover, relatively well-traveled mental paths also appear to be more likely to be activated; once established and reinforced, the well-worn road invites more future travel than less explored paths.

In light of our brain architecture, we can expect that our process of remembering is vulnerable to the prompts and reinforcements that everyday conversation provides on a regular basis. Although interpersonal sources are objectively different from a television sitcom, interacting with another person may affect our memory for that television show. Every time we entertain interpersonal communication, our behavior should arouse at least some related content in our brains, including representations of mass media content previously encoded and formed.

Once we look at people in this way, audiences for mass media messages become more complicated. Rather than seeing people as stand-alone addresses for information delivery and encoding, we can view people as being interconnected pieces of a larger community that, in turn, may need to be addressed as a whole because of the potential for interpersonal exchange to impact campaign message reception. For example, general conversation about the specific public health dangers of hurricanes, flooding, or earthquakes could reinforce or amplify memory for connected material gleaned from mass media reports on those topics. The same is true for LED light bulbs. Interpersonal communication about the actual media content in question could also reinforce memory for that content. Simple conversation about news stories facilitates the long-term storage and retrieval of information from those stories.[15] Talking to others may pave the way for our long-term memory or forgetting.

In my research on memory measurement, I found multiple instances in which conversations act as echo chambers and amplifying stations to boost the salience of ideas to which people were exposed previously. In one example,[16] colleagues and I conducted a series of in-depth interviews with a group of adults around the United States to begin to understand prevalent conceptions of "science" and "scientists." The original interview protocol included a plan to talk with people in a focus group format, meaning they would talk together with a group of other participants and a moderator. We wanted to know how often the news and entertainment programming each person recently viewed directly referred to scientists or science. In order to ask people about that mass media content, we needed to decide when we were going to ask them about what science-related content they remembered recently seeing—either before or after they had an otherwise wide-ranging discussion with other participants about a variety of ideas. Consequently, we embedded an experiment into the study to assess whether the discussion with other participants might matter. We randomly assigned the participants into one of two groups and had both groups fill out a questionnaire both before and after the peer discussion. One group's questionnaire included a question about their memory of recent media content, whereas the other half was assigned a questionnaire that did not include that question. We then allowed the discussions to take place and administered a second questionnaire. For the questionnaire given *after* the discussion, those participants whose initial questionnaire included the memory question completed a version of the questionnaire without that question, whereas those who had not initially been assigned to answer the memory question were given a questionnaire that included the question. In other words, everyone answered the same memory question, but one group did so without having been exposed to the discussion with others and the other group did so only immediately after discussion.

One might expect that generally the order of the questions would not make a difference. In all cases, after all, participants were asked to respond about mass media exposure that ostensibly had occurred prior to the interviews. One may presume that whether participants answered just before or just after participation in the group discussion should not affect the fidelity of their memory for recent mass media mentions of science. However, participants assigned to talk with others about science immediately prior to reporting memory of television mentions of science were *four times* more likely to report recent mass media mentions than participants in the control condition ($p < .01$). Interpersonal discussion, the only factor randomly assigned to differ between people, appears to have amplified basic memory. Most likely, the discussions with others prompted neural nodes that had been largely dormant just prior to the discussions. In other words, talk with other people about science and scientists made *all* science-related content more *salient* and consequently more easily retrievable.

Evidence from a national survey of adolescents about their attitudes toward drug use and their memory of anti-drug advertisements produced and aired by the White House offers a consistent picture. In that study,[9] conversation with friends and family members appears to have enhanced the salience of advertising. A teenager's simple memory of an advertisement appears to have been reinforced or diminished as a function of talk with others in their social network. Figure 2 illustrates the basic pattern suggested in that study: living amidst an active set of conversations about a topic enhanced memory for advertisements about that topic.

Figure 2. Talk in social networks and the translation of advertisement exposure into memory

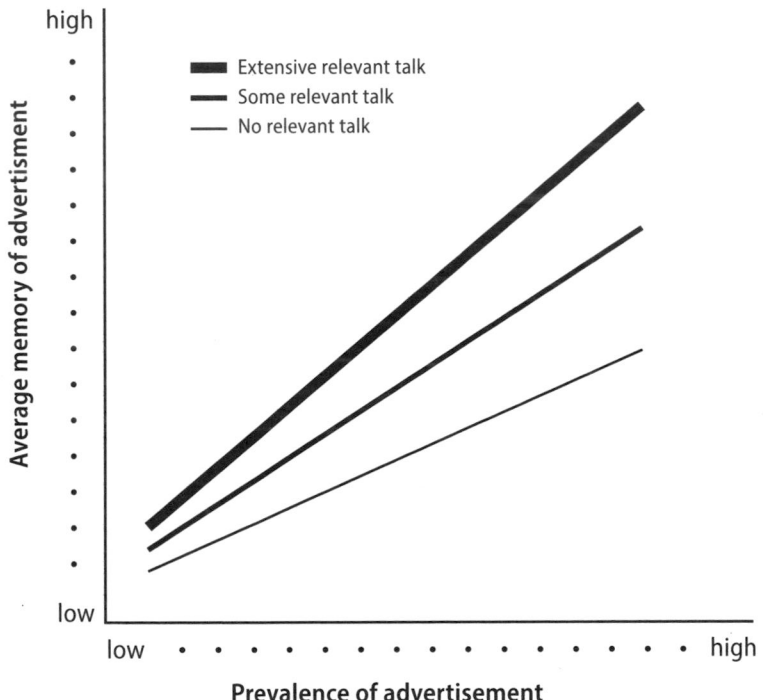

How exactly did conversation enhance memory of advertisements? The amount of relevant conversation in a respondent's environment interacted with the sheer prevalence of an advertisement in a person's television market and helped to explain recognition memory for that advertisement. Using a combination of advertisement purchasing data and survey data, I found a positive relationship between the frequency and reach of an anti-drug advertisement on television—measured in terms of what advertisers call purchased or earned "gross ratings points" for an advertisement—and the degree to which people later remembered viewing that advertisement. The extent to which television market advertisement prevalence translated into individual memory, however, depended on whether a person reported living in a social network that was abundant with conversation about drugs. People who often engaged in relevant conversation about drugs also tended to be those who later remembered prevalent campaign advertisements, beyond what would be expected based simply on their other characteristics.

One way of conceptualizing this type of effect is as *enhancement* (or dampening) of the effects of a campaign. Conversation or other forms of social interaction may be a result of exposure to media content. Nonetheless, such interaction may sometimes amplify or dampen the effects that mass media exposure otherwise would have. Such an effect is what social scientists call *variable interaction* or *moderation*.[17]

Inasmuch as brain performance could be vulnerable to our social network interactions is likely an uncomfortable realization for many of us. As Carr[18] noted, "we have a sense that our brain exists in a state of splendid isolation, that its fundamental nature is impervious to the vagaries of our day-to-day lives" (p. 38). In the case of our daily interactions with others, it appears that chitchat matters. It can affect what is on our mind, in the colloquial sense, and can impact what of the information torrent becomes driftwood and what sinks far below the surface. The fact that such a powerful filter of our recent reality resides in what otherwise seems to be an innocuous conversation with one's aunt gives us yet another reason to pay attention to the networks in which we live.

Social Norm Awareness

Another effect of social network interaction involves the unleashing of normative pressure. Certainly, conversations and social interaction allow a wide range of information diffusion, and talk between people does more than simply communicate social norms.[19] Nonetheless, prompting conversation and interaction with other people can lead to learning about what others think about your behavior and learning about what it is that others do. That may have an encouraging or discouraging effect on your intentions, beyond what you personally thought about your plans prior to the conversation. Imagine proudly announcing your intention to start commuting to work by bicycle, only to have your friend express concerns about safety on the roads or the impracticality of your showing up at work hot and sweaty. Moreover, imagine how you might feel if that friend simply looked blankly at you as though you had said something odd and then promptly changed the subject.

Hornik and Yanovitzky[20] attempted to outline various ways that media campaigns that are intended to change human behavior operate. Consistent with the present argument, they stressed that campaign exposure may lead a person to talk with others about campaign messages and to discover normative support (or lack thereof). By acting as a conversational prompt, a campaign could lead people to find out that others support particular behaviors more than one may have originally supposed. The net impact is indirect encouragement of behavior change via social norms.

Empirical evidence from the global public health literature supports this idea. Evaluation of a contraceptive promotion campaign in Bolivia in the 1990s, for example, highlighted a positive link between media campaign exposure and change over time in the perception that other people in particular social networks actually use contraceptives.[21,22] This potential norm discovery or enhancement effect echoes Hornik and Yanovitzky's contentions and suggests that audience members for a campaign will vary in their ultimate outcomes as a function of variance in the network norms they discover around them.

Work by Durkin and Wakefield[23] on tobacco cessation is another example of how discussions may activate normative influence. These researchers studied smokers in Australia who were shown anti-tobacco advertisements. After showing participants the advertisements, Durkin and Wakefield used a follow-up survey to track whether participants talked with others about the anti-smoking advertising after seeing it. They found that having talked with others did not significantly impact participants' personal concern about their own smoking. Participants who interacted with others after seeing the ad, however, were more likely to report that they intended to quit. In other words, talking with others did not necessarily appear to affect one's attitude toward smoking as a personal matter, but it did appear to activate normative pressure. An example conversation comes from a mother in the study who, when asked what she actually discussed with others, reported simply, "My daughters hassled me to give up smoking … they hate it" (p. 8).

Crucially, the possibility for norm activation is very much a double-edged sword. Activating networks can be the equivalent of stirring a hornet's nest. Consider the work of David, Cappella, and Fishbein[24] to understand the effects anti-drug public service announcements on teenagers. These researchers found that chat between people *negatively* affected the persuasive impact of advertising intended to reduce adolescent substance use.

David and colleagues illustrated how interpersonal communication can undermine, rather than facilitate, campaign persuasion goals. Importantly, their account depends on the availability of supportive or denigrating people as conversational partners. This study used an innovative design not only to randomly assign people to see the advertising in question, but also to capture the conversation that followed using one of the technologies discussed in Chapter 3. The study assigned some participants to chat with other participants in an online chat forum following exposure to the anti-drug campaign advertisements. Group discussion apparently unfolded and functioned in a way not anticipated by the campaign planners. Participants who had been assigned to talk with others actually reported attitudes and normative beliefs that were more strongly in favor of marijuana use than their counterparts who simply watched the ads and were not assigned to use the chat function to talk with anyone about the ads.

What happened here? David and colleagues smartly assessed who actually tended to participate in the online chats. They discovered that the individuals who were most likely to engage the anti-drug ads in a biased fashion—those who believed strongly that marijuana use was enjoyable—also tended to be people who contributed to group discussions, which skewed the chats that followed. Many of the comments in the group discussions depicted drug use positively. Consequently, participants who lurked on the sidelines of such chat actually heard numerous pro-drug viewpoints. It appears that exposure to the chat affected both attitudinal and normative perceptions: people were hearing arguments in favor of drug use, and were hearing such arguments from live people similar in age and background to themselves. Evidence supports this interpretation, as people who were experimentally assigned to discuss the ads subsequently reported more normative pressure to use marijuana following the conversations than did people who only saw the ads in isolation.

Consequently, discussion can be an uncooperative partner at times for advertising campaign planners and strategic communication professionals. Even if a campaign manages to generate conversation, campaign staff cannot guarantee that the resulting talk will coincide with campaign goals, especially when many of the individuals viewing the campaign have reason for substantial bias in their interpretation of campaign materials. For that reason, all advertising campaigns, both those that explicitly strive to spark conversation and those that do not, have at least some reason for caution. Regardless, social norms seem likely to be more prominent and more frequently reinforced among people living in actively chattering networks compared with people living in relative solitude and isolation.

Conferral of Argument Resistance

Compton and Pfau[25] discovered an intriguing result when they attempted to inoculate college students against credit card marketing. By actively presenting both sides of an argument regarding credit card initiation rather than simply presenting a one-sided argument against credit cards, these researchers were able to reduce student vulnerability to subsequent credit card marketing. (They call this strategy inoculation, a communication approach that draws inspiration from the medical inoculation model: instead of exposing people to a weakened virus as a way of increasing resistance to the live virus, audiences are exposed to two sides of an argument in an effort to promote resistance to one side of the argument.) Most important for our discussion is the fact that students who received the inoculation message reportedly also intended to warn their friends of the dangers of credit cards. That is, they were less likely to tout the positive benefits of credit cards and more likely to discuss the negative potential. These results suggested that perhaps social networks can be a vector for the spread of inoculation.

Compton and Pfau[26] further developed the notion that social interaction can help to confer resistance to future persuasion attempts, whether it be fast food marketing or offering of illicit drugs. Not only did they suggest that two-sided messages may increase the likelihood of people subsequently discussing the message, in part due to the uncertainty that such an approach introduces, they also argued that interaction between people can introduce people to multiple sides of an argument.

Consider the example of LED light bulb adoption introduced earlier in this chapter. Imagine that a woman, inspired by information about the pros and cons of LED bulbs to not only adopt the new light bulbs but also to promote them, turns to others in an attempt to promote their use of LED bulbs. She may run into some resistance. When she wants to replace all of the bulbs in her house with LED bulbs, her outspoken partner may protest, for example, by saying that he does not like the aesthetic appearance of the light cast by LED light bulbs. It may take some effort to sharpen the argument in favor of LED bulb adoption before the woman is ultimately successful in converting their entire household. That trial by fire, however, may embolden and empower the woman to talk with additional skeptical neighbors and friends because now she has been exposed to counterarguments and has a set of available responses to challenges. Further, when the incandescent bulb marketers attempt to lure this woman back to the cheaper incandescent bulbs, the conversational activity within her social network may help to steel her against the persuasion. A person living among a less active network may enjoy less of that empowerment against future countermarketing.

The Consequences of Social Network Interaction

Theoretically, all of these information-sharing outcomes—knowledge gain, cognitive salience, social norm awareness, and conferral of argument resistance—are potential accelerants, if not necessarily main causes, of intergroup disparities in health behavior, civic activity, and even collective decision-making. That is not to say that the ripple effects of such social network activation hold uniform valence. Unleashing forces such as social norms or resistance to arguments clearly could operate in multiple ways depending on the exact nature of the norms or the arguments in question. Increasing the salience of unhealthy norms or conferring resistance to messages intended to improve well-being, for example, may be unwelcome effects, and we may be grateful that some groups are shielded from such effects by having reduced access to conversations.

Also, not all of these consequences are likely to be equally important. Differences in knowledge gain about nuclear fusion, for example, may not impact a person's everyday life as much as awareness of the latest asthma guidelines. Being reminded of the general advantages of renewable energy sources may not be as consequential for a person's energy conservation behavior as becoming more aware of what neighbors think about a person actually installing solar power panels on a house. Nonetheless, based on our review of potential consequences of increased interpersonal interaction, it is clear that gaps between people may widen through a variety of mechanisms and that in many instances that disparity in interaction ultimately could undermine healthy behavior or popular engagement with scientific research.

Consider obesity. Undoubtedly, the obesity epidemic that unfolded in the United States in the late 20th century had various root causes, including the corn-based economy of the nation.[27] Differences between people in their experience of obesity also have been affected by structural factors, such as the lack of nutritious, relatively less fattening food in many neighborhood stores.[28] At the same time, all four of the aforementioned information-sharing consequences—knowledge gain, cognitive salience, social norm awareness, and conferral of argument resistance—may have played either a facilitating or inhibiting role in indirectly widening the gaps between people in terms of their body mass index (BMI).

The Internet is full of information about diet and physical activity recommendations that can assist a person in maintaining a healthy BMI. (Of course, the Internet is overflowing with less helpful advice as well.) A person's careful perusal of such information on her or his own could be met, regularly, with either reinforcing or distracting interactions with others. Moreover, some of the discussion a person might encounter could involve outright mockery. Consider the path of the lonely vegetarian who is mocked by family for eating, literally, like a bird. Posting about day one of a new diet on ones's Facebook page may bring surprising and welcome support from others, discouraging ridicule, or, perhaps most disconcerting, absolutely no response at all. Insofar as the availability of supportive interpersonal interactions is a function of social advantage and status, we can see how some people may end up more vulnerable to obesity than others in a disparate way.

Evaluation research by Richardson and colleagues[29] to assess the impact of an intervention intended to promote walking as a pathway toward healthy weight provides direct empirical support of the general idea that engagement with social networks can reinforce or undermine health outcomes. This study found that having access to an online support community positively affected participants' adherence to the program. People who had online support— support that was randomly assigned in a carefully controlled experiment— ultimately were more successful in participating in the program over time. Without access to support from others, participation waned, relatively speaking.

One way of envisioning the possibilities that the social network tendencies afford, or at least privilege, for information flow is to picture a rectangular board and a marble. If we assume the board to be perfectly flat, then rolling the marble will lead to a predictable path of progress. Any holes or bumps in the board, however, will complicate our prediction of the marble's path. One might consider an overlay of social networks to act as something of a pinball machine relative to broadcast information, amplifying the trajectory of some information and allowing other information to fall silent.

Moody and White[30] offered another direct metaphor when they discussed the impact of variability in the social cohesion of groups. They noted that "local pockets of high connectivity act as amplifying substations for information (or resource, or viral) flow that comes into the more highly connected group, boosting a signal's strength … and sending it back out into the wider population" (p. 120). From this perspective, it is the underlying *unevenness* of network connectivity that matters as a conditioning force, not simply the fact that people can be connected to one another and share information. Some types of information that enter small groups will get amplified in volume beyond what may be expected, whereas information that has no path into a group will fall silent.

What type of information we are considering, who is involved in passing along (or not passing along) that information, and how people are connected to others all play a role in shaping what is on our mind on any given day. As discussed in this chapter, it is not simply the verbatim transfer of a message from one person to another that can be affected. Unevenness in the networks available to a person can affect whether that person is regularly reminded of key ideas or even whether she or he engages information in a deep way, such as developing resistance to arguments over time. Individuals who have the benefit of active networks of friends, family members, and colleagues who constantly discuss and share the latest information on how to eat in a healthy way or how to conserve household energy appear to enjoy all kinds of regular support in thinking deeply about those topics themselves. At the same time, unevenness in the connections available to people—unevenness that is not necessarily chosen and maybe not what people would choose if they could—can translate into differences between people in their daily *engagement* with information and not just in their exposure to new information. In other words, unevenness in social network activity also means that some people spend more time deeply considering (or even just being reminded of) information than others. Among the consequences of information-sharing disparities are varying degrees of salience and contemplation, and not simply new information exposure. What is on one's mind much of the time is subject to the talking and sharing that surrounds a person in everyday life.

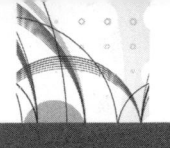

CHAPTER 8

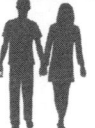

Remedies and Realism

Throughout this book, I have argued that a broad array of social science literature supports the contention that information that diffuses interpersonally will not spread uniformly across large populations. Social ties between some people and the absence of such ties will leave some people less likely than others to hear about new ideas related to human health and scientific research. Moreover, the volume, topic, and nature of everyday chatter that surrounds people appear to vary dramatically between them. Despite enthusiasm about 21st century possibilities for social contagion as a mechanism for public education, we have distinct reasons to expect not only inequality but also inequity. Whether and how to address such disparity are questions we have not yet directly addressed, and a thorough consideration of what might be done to tackle the issues raised throughout this book will not be complete unless we do so.

Why Are Information-Sharing Disparities Problematic?

The question of intervention invites a set of ethical considerations. In pursuing answers to this question, it is useful to acknowledge the inevitability of failure in attempting to please all readers on this dimension. Many current political debates signal core ideological differences between people in the extent to which they value collective well-being and equity versus protection of individual liberty regardless of society's collective needs. Such debates will not be solved here, but instead we can outline factors that seem amenable to certain types of change and suggest what can be done to address some of the patterns discussed in this book for those concerned about them.

In considering whether to worry about information-sharing differences, some people may ask whether ultimately it would be useful or appropriate to somehow distribute knowledge uniformly throughout society. Importantly, we have discussed much more than just the verbatim *dissemination* of information from person to person in considering interpersonal interaction, so information distribution is not the only criterion to raise. We may also worry about equal opportunities for deliberation or for prompts and reminders. In raising concerns about all sorts of information-sharing inequalities, I nonetheless have begged the question of *why* we should care about such inequality at all. Amartya Sen, writing in *Inequality Reexamined*,[1] noted that any useful ethical consideration of equality must address two questions: "Why equality?" and "Equality of what?" Consequently, in this case we must take a look at why equal access to information-sharing efforts by other people should be valued. The case for focusing on equality as a general virtue seems defensible, as Sen noted that "every normative theory of social arrangement that has at all stood the test of time seems to demand equality of *something*" (p. 12). Yet why ensuring that we all are regularly and actively reached by colleagues, friends, or family with efforts to share information about the health effects of wine or with neuroscience research on attraction is not as clear.

Some even will argue that all people do not need to be equally engaged with science information, let alone information *sharing*, because in-depth understanding of specialized topics is not necessary for collective decision-making. Certainly, that is the essential line of thinking that animated arguments by Lippmann[2,3] for the inevitability of a national population in the United States that always will be divided into an active audience and the remaining unengaged. Traces of that thinking appear in more recent commentary on the prospects for science communication. Nisbet and Scheufele[4] argued that basic efforts to educate a "wider public" beyond science enthusiasts simply are not promising, as most people have little appetite, or day-to-day need, for scientific information. Importantly, they also argued that worrying about simple differences in the sheer amount of technical scientific knowledge people hold is not even productive, as people often make decisions about funding and support for science based on heuristics and their personal values. Variance in the salience of, and engagement with, particular issues undoubtedly matters to them, but incomplete diffusion of detailed technical knowledge may not be a dire circumstance.

The specific case of health information may seem more difficult to address with such an argument because in many instances individuals need information to make well-informed decisions that influence their personal health. Nonetheless, the average person likely does not need not to hold an advanced medical degree or a graduate degree in public health to understand enough about the benefits of a cancer screening or regular physical activity to act in a way that will improve their well-being. Consequently, it is possible to even plausibly argue that some despair and concern over health information-sharing disparities is superfluous by suggesting that there is a ceiling point beyond which gaps and disparities are inconsequential.

Nonetheless, now is a prime moment to recall our initial distinction between differences and disparities. The preceding chapters offered evidence highlighting the tendency of people to vary in their preponderance of peer-to-peer engagement regarding science and health. Admittedly, not all of that variance in peer-to-peer engagement is similarly likely to inspire intervention. The fact that some people who have the opportunity and are free to choose to share information with their family and friends (and to benefit from such sharing) opt not to do so is likely best viewed as little more than a guarantee of discourse diversity. Some of the factors that appear to predict communicative differences seem tied to personality or individual preferences in ways that underscore inequality but do not necessarily beg consideration of injustice. Other factors, however, especially those discussed in Chapter 5 focusing on community-level differences, signal potential disparity that arguably suggests troubling inequity between people that could be avoided with effort and is beyond what we might choose if given the choice.

In worrying about individual- and community-level differences that seem largely outside of a person's everyday control, we do not have to simply argue for the inherent value of equal information distribution to make a case for intervening to overcome information-sharing disparities. Two major considerations warrant acknowledgment in this regard. One involves the role of peer-to-peer sharing as a potentially vital supplement to our everyday information diet, whereas the other involves our 21st century temptation to assume that technology is connecting people in revolutionary fashion when it is not doing so uniformly.

With regard to the first consideration, as discussed throughout the book, peer-to-peer information sharing is often an unsolicited source of prompting from other people. Without that prompting and sharing, we are each left largely with the information we seek and engage on our own. While the Internet provides theoretical access to an overwhelming array of information to many, we can only expect most people to engage a small sliver of that information on their own each day. So, we cannot depend on individual behavior alone to compensate for network-level tendencies.

As to the second consideration, one of the major reasons why information-sharing disparities are problematic is that their existence is now relatively easy to overlook by those who are ensconced in social networks that regularly buzz with activity. In other words, *a major reason to worry about the disparity patterns documented in this book is that many people increasingly are tempted to assume that they do not exist.* That leaves many of us with an incomplete picture of the information engagement of fellow citizens and people around the world. If we evaluate the state of consumer decision-making regarding health behavior or citizen support for scientific research and assume that it reflects a society in which everyone is not only constantly seeking information on their own but also fully enjoying a rich bounty of shared information, then we may make decisions based on a faulty view. Even if one does not agree that access to peer-to-peer communication regarding health and science ought to be standardized, those who value accuracy at least should agree that correcting a faulty view of our "networked" society is worthwhile.

It is also important to remember that not all of the information-sharing disparities that might motivate concern lie in the differences between individual people or even between communities. Some of those differences actually affect us collectively and could concern us for additional reasons. By simply talking about some issues more than others, we habitually remind ourselves of those issues more than others. Therefore, the salience of those ideas may stem, in part, from differences in the nature of media content to generate more or less interpersonal interaction. One of the implications of the discussion in Chapter 6 about message-level factors is that collectively we may be predisposed to share certain types of information repeatedly and rarely to amplify the signal of others. Together we are circulating less of the information than perhaps we would if we somehow could prioritize our discussions to focus on, for example, scientific advancements to improve the suitability of the global environment for endangered species.

How Can Disparities Be Remedied?

For those who see value in encouraging greater information sharing between people in particular populations or communities, several paths toward intervention are apparent in light of the evidence presented in this book. While some degree of inequality in information sharing is inevitable, we can strive to eliminate inequitable disparities in three major ways: boosting collective confidence, meeting people where they are, and building the connection infrastructure available to those in question.

Boost Collective Confidence

We know that people are not particularly likely to share information they do not think they understand. Absent direct encouragement to challenge or engage with scientific ideas, such as research on medical innovations or biotechnology, many people will silently defer to those they see as relatively expert.[5] Moreover, as we have seen with research on the role of perceived understanding in prompting conversation and information sharing, there are numerous reasons why confidence in one's own understanding is crucial.[6,7] Individuals who feel as though they can grasp key ideas are more likely to subsequently share those ideas with others.

Beyond the confidence any one individual has or may gain, we also can start to think about the collective confidence that may or may not be embedded in groups. The extent to which multiple people in a community have a sense of understanding is likely predictive ultimately of whether people in that group feel as though they can seek information from others and discuss relevant information with others. In other words, a productive strategy may be not only to attempt to make scientific information more accessible to individuals but also to address groups.

This strategy is apparent in the work, for example, of an organization called Clean Energy Durham, a 501(c)(3) nonprofit founded in North Carolina that produces training products and services under the brand name Pete Street. One of their key slogans is "Where Neighbors Get Energy Savings." Former Executive Director Judy Kincaid described their approach as one focused on neighborhoods and peer-to-peer information sharing within neighborhoods. This organization advises groups of neighbors together at the same time on energy-saving tips and ideas. The collective address is important so that when any one person in the group wants to act but cannot remember exactly how to implement a particular tip, that person can rely on the collective memory of her or his neighborhood peers. Whether to find out the best way to clean a refrigerator, change light bulbs, or implement a full energy retrofit, neighbors can learn from each other even after the trainer has left the scene.

What is innovative about Clean Energy Durham's strategy is that they do not solely depend on individuals who learn about energy facts to turn and share them with their neighbors and family members. Expecting widespread information sharing without carefully considering the network infrastructure for collaboration in a community is a recipe for fizzling rather than viral explosion. By addressing groups of neighbors together at the same time, organizations like Clean Energy Durham are making energy savings a salient topic for community collaboration and offering the type of topical knowledge and vocabulary to facilitate neighbor-to-neighbor information sharing that appears to be at least one remedy to some of the concerns outlined in this book.

Meet People Where They Are

Earlier, I noted that ideas appear most likely to enter everyday discourse when they somehow resonate with people's daily routines and concerns. This suggests that those who are strategically hoping to spark peer-to-peer information sharing need to understand the everyday lives of the people among whom they hope messages and ideas will spread. In other words, strategic efforts to leverage social networks that attempt to introduce ideas largely askance to the rhythm and flow of daily conversation are likely to sink without much dissemination.

Within science communication circles, the notion of framing ideas in popular terms intersects with a long-standing debate that centers precisely on the question of whether science needs to be understood by everyone and whether using metaphors and examples that are widely understood but perhaps not completely accurate is appropriate. Some science educators have pursued popularization efforts that attempt to spread scientific knowledge developed by scientists to wider audiences in simplified form.[8] Informal science education efforts, in turn, have been met with critique, claiming that popularization oversimplifies how scientific knowledge should function in a society.[8,9] Logan,[9] for example, called for citizens to be involved in the discourse necessary to develop scientific findings relevant to society and to resolve emergent concerns. Whether involving citizens in regular institutional decision-making is feasible is an important question. Even aside from formal involvement in decision-making processes, there are opportunities to frame ongoing scientific challenges in everyday language. Technical communication professionals are very familiar with this task, as their work involves the science of making complex information accessible, usable, and relevant to a variety of audiences.[10]

Nisbet and Scheufele[11] embraced the need to essentially frame scientific findings in ways that resonate with the needs and interests of different audiences. As they noted, even Google cofounder Larry Page said that "science has a serious marketing problem" (p. 39). What they suggested is that emergent issues in science, such as nanotechnology or stem cell research, should be presented in a way that fits the predominant interests of the audience in question: "For example, when scientists are speaking to … people who think about the world primarily in economic terms, they should emphasize the economic relevance of science—such as, in the case of embryonic stem cell research, pointing out that expanded government funding would make the United States, or a particular state, more economically competitive" (p. 39).

Build Community Connection Infrastructure

People need to be connected to others if they are to share information with them or to benefit from such sharing. Without available community ties, as we have seen, efforts to promote peer referral falter. How to build community connections is a large question. Moreover, simply building a set of mutually interlocking connections between members of a small group without facilitating any connection to people outside of the group is a recipe for high levels of trust within the group but relatively little prospect for helpful information to enter that closed loop of people. How can we build connection infrastructure in a way that prepares communities for future opportunities for information sharing?

As a start, we can look toward different conceptualizations of community now afforded by new communication technologies. Technology now makes available online forums regarding particular topics that may offer some remedy for the gaps in network resources discussed throughout this book. Payton and colleagues[12] discussed the utility of connecting African-American female college students interested in information related to HIV through a Web-based portal and hub. Horner[13] examined interactions among a group of parents brought together by their children's diagnoses of fragile X syndrome, a genetically transmitted disease affecting mental and emotional abilities. Similarly, Rupert and colleagues[14] investigated the experiences of members of online discussion forums hosted by PatientsLikeMe.com and WebMD.

Assessment of the experiences of group members offers a mix of encouragement and discouragement. Horner[13] followed the actual online proceedings of a group of parents connected by an e-mail listserv maintained by a national research funding organization for fragile X syndrome. Among that group, apparently only some actively and regularly contributed, as many subscribers largely lurked, meaning they read but rarely contributed. Nonetheless, the forum appears to offer a resource for connection. While the group served political purposes—to organize advocacy for additional fragile X funding—members also connected with one another to offer support and advice. Consequently, the group represents a virtual network and community that likely facilitated information sharing beyond what otherwise would have existed in members' lives.

Rupert and collaborators[14] talked with verified members of online health communities and found that many members joined a discussion group after receiving a major medical diagnosis. Members tended to seek information about treatment options, what to expect during medical appointments, and illness details. What members appeared to offer and share with one another is telling. Overall, members were more likely to share their personal treatment experiences than to forward wholesale factual treatment information. The forums appear to be places for bonding, connection, and social support more than for inquiry as to the latest scientific findings.

Importantly, these groups do not always simply facilitate and deliver social support. Horner's study of a fragile X advocacy group highlights tensions in group discourse and defections by members over time as various members discussed sensitive issues, such as the extent to which disabled children can or should be expected to somehow contribute to society as they age in return for legal protections. Nonetheless, group moderators interested in promoting supportive environments may be able to assess intragroup conflict and help to at least ensure civility.

Also noteworthy is the fact that online support groups can arise organically in response to a variety of topics and issues in ways that are not carefully planned. Additionally, the predominant tone and perspective of subsequent conversations may not always be in line with that of public health officials or professional scientists. Consider research on a pro-anorexia online discussion forum.[15] Over time, postings suggested support for member's identification with anorexia as a positive part of their identity and also suggested bonding among group members over time. Cases like this one present an important, if complex, set of ideas. Arguably, group members in such dialogue gain a sense of camaraderie that can reduce social isolation. However, the existence of the created network can encourage what many medical professionals would call markedly unhealthy behavior.

Online forums also undoubtedly can fuel the flames of controversy. Consider online discussion of the so-called Climategate incident. In late 2009, e-mail exchanges between prominent climate scientists in the United Kingdom regarding debate over research results were published on the Internet and subsequently used by conservative bloggers as evidence of the fallibility of the argument for humans' role in climate change. Nerlich[16] argued that blog postings complaining about the e-mails led mass media news coverage by at least a week and played an important role in bolstering the sense of controversy.

Nonetheless, active efforts to connect people to one another, such as the PatientsLikeMe health information system, appear to facilitate disease self-management and provide a sense of support otherwise lacking for patients.[17] It is likely that a similar effort could promote energy conservation or pro-environment behavior. Moreover, Cobb, Graham, and Abrams[18] showed that a network stemming from the active construction of an online community, such as the smoking cessation group QuitNet, can look similar to offline social networks that endure over time and harbor active communication among various group members, rather than simply representing broadcast of messages from a single source to an audience.

Perhaps one key to building community connections is to avoid assuming that wholesale new community construction is the right path to pursue. Perhaps there are ways to bolster and improve connection infrastructure in already existent spaces. At least one scholar who is optimistic about the possibilities afforded by new communication technologies offered an approach refreshingly grounded in, rather than aspiring to transcend beyond, place. Keith Hampton is among those who have argued that the introduction of Internet-based networking technology may help to alleviate previous gaps in connectivity among relatively disadvantaged groups. For example, Hampton[19] wrote that the Internet appears capable of affording civic engagement in contexts that historically have been characterized by extreme disadvantage. He reported on experience with the *i-Neighbors* project, which allowed neighborhoods to have access to Internet-based resources that facilitated local interaction. As Hampton pointed out, *i-Neighbors* communities in his study corresponded to actual geographic communities dispersed over thousands of US zip codes. Visitors to the *i-Neighbors* website could create an account, join a digital version of their own geographic neighborhood, and communicate and share information with those neighbors, assuming at least some other residents of their neighborhood joined. In analyzing evidence of interaction among users, Hampton found that many of the most active neighborhoods were in census tracts located in relatively disadvantaged areas.

A posted message from one of the participants in Hampton's study illustrates the apparent possibilities when connection infrastructure is built:

> Before, people would call me with information that I knew needed to be spread around, but I did not have the tools to do it and it was frustrating.… We have a powerful way to communicate with each other whenever we need to.… We have caught criminals and … given out tips for securing our homes; removed a postal carrier from our neighborhood who drank on the job…; created lasting friendships; cleaned up our streets; recommended neighbors who are skilled craftspeople to each other; found homes for stray animals; fixed water leaks; kept each other informed of important neighborhood news…; and, yes, even vented some frustration. (p. 1128)

What seems to be crucial in Hampton's approach is the marriage of locally based networks with connective technologies. The solution appears not to be an attempt to simply transcend place and location, as geography undoubtedly continues to matter. By affording connections between neighbors and people with shared geographical interests, projects such as those described by Hampton have the potential to build functional relationships that are more useful than the myriad but ephemeral ties that seem available purely online.

Importantly, a key aspect of Hampton's approach, beyond its acknowledgment that geography matters, is the *provision* of Internet access to those without it. This suggests we cannot overlook the basic importance of technology access as a part of the story of information flow. Major gaps in high-speed Internet access remain in the United States and elsewhere, whether considering disparities between rural and urban residents or between different socioeconomic groups.[20,21]

Some aspects of the communication technology picture are changing. Kontos and colleagues[21] reported that among Internet users, neither socioeconomic status nor race and ethnicity predicted differences in social networking site use, meaning that some historically underserved groups now are gravitating toward social media use in similar fashion to other groups once they have basic technology access. Nonetheless, even widespread enthusiasm for social media use among Internet users masks some continued underlying discrepancies. In the Kontos et al. study, for example, adults with cancer were less likely to have used a social networking site than others, even after age and other demographic factors were controlled. In other words, enthusiasm for technology-based solutions to equalizing opportunities for health and science flow needs to be tempered by acknowledgment of the real differences in technology access and use that currently exist.

In the realm of emergency management, White[22] recently championed the potential for building connections between people using technological remedies as an active plan to promote community preparedness. She claimed that crowdsourcing as an approach to surveillance makes sense because "citizens are the greatest resource of untapped information right now" (p. 47). By ensuring connections between people, we can encourage information sharing by a broad array of individuals, which will assist not only in boosting the spread of preparedness training information but also in mapping victim locations and disseminating information during an actual emergency response.

White also admitted, however, that simply introducing any sort of connective technology will not ensure the sort of functional connections that are necessary. On a basic level, we should worry about the vulnerability of social media (as computer-dependent tools) to power disruptions, software glitches, and other technological failures. Individuals attempting to use social media on the New Jersey coast during the peak of Hurricane Sandy in 2012 needed at least cell phone power to do so. White also suggested that not all technology remedies are equal. She recommended using what she calls user-focused applications that afford some user control over content posting and rely on open-source software that allows multiple authors to fix problems and for the application to evolve over time to fit user needs. In comparing several contemporary social media applications, for example, she trumpeted the relative ease of searching Twitter feeds relative to the difficulty of finding relevant posts on Facebook. If the goal is allowing institutions and individuals to quickly see calls for help, practical tips posted by individuals, and the latest information updates from officials, people need transparent applications that allow them to look for information posted by others. In other words, social media applications that encourage closed-off pockets and groups of people who talk only to one another are less useful than applications promoting a large number of available ties or connections across a geographic community for whom emergency-related information is relevant.

Acknowledging Disparities While Moving Forward

Part of the goal in introducing the ideas in this book is purely pragmatic: to document a paradox about the value of peer-to-peer strategies that tend to be overlooked by many communication professionals. That intention should not be confused with simple dismissal of peer-to-peer communication efforts. Contemporary interest in peer-to-peer strategies makes sense at first glance. Some strategies in that vein hold promise to extend program reach in a relatively inexpensive way, and the possibilities for *involving* audiences rather than just broadcasting *to* them will be appealing for many projects. People involved in educating large masses of people about the latest research on topics like healthy behavior or the natural environment do not typically have access to bullhorns that can reach everyone at once. Numerous factors constrain communication professionals, particularly those working for nonprofit institutions, including our increasingly fragmented mass media landscape, the sheer cost of mass media advertising, and institutional norms among news outlets that can make generating news coverage difficult for nonprofit organizations. These and other barriers make reaching large populations at once difficult. Consequently, some have considered person-to-person alternatives to spread the words they wish to spread, leveraging the myriad relationships and connections between people that undoubtedly are available. Others have hoped to spark public dialogue in the same fashion by seeding social networks with information they hope will encourage discussion. Nonetheless, relying on peer-to-peer information sharing brings its own limitations, despite the changes witnessed in recent years with regard to social media technologies.

In this regard, hyperbole about a supposed social media revolution is not useful, as changes in communication technology have not eliminated the interpersonal interaction differences that abound in our nation and around the world, even as the pace of change has quickened and technology has made some types of interactions more possible than was the case decades ago. Despite new technologies, people continue to vary in their personal resources for connecting with one another; communities vary as well. Moreover, as we have discussed, most people simply do not take advantage of readily available opportunities they have to pass information along to anyone else. When measured across everyone who is initially exposed to broadcast information, subsequent peer-to-peer referral generally appears to be the exception rather than the rule, despite the fact that some content does "go viral."

Consequently, presenting information to an initial audience cannot be expected to result in a uniform spread outward from that group to the rest of a society in a perfect set of concentric circles like ripples in a pond. We are organized and live in information environments that are much rougher and more nuanced than the glassy surface of a body of water. Some of the roughness—the grouping of people into cliques and networks from which some people are excluded—reflects disparities that are lamentable if one cares about equality between people. Some of the roughness simply reflects a healthy diversity of interests and habits among people. Diversity of viewpoints, of course, is useful for debate. However, the flowering of deliberation among informed citizens, in an ideal sense, is less likely in circumstances in which people do not have ready and willing conversational partners through which to get information they otherwise would not have received and with whom to develop and test ideas. Absent careful planning beforehand, simple reliance on peer-to-peer information-sharing strategies will not automatically eliminate, and may even reify, information disparities between people and will not necessarily generate widespread public dialogue.

Over and above encouraging pragmatic acceptance of our current prospects for organizing and orchestrating peer-to-peer communication, this discussion has offered some measure of justification and hope for those who wish to address any of the sharing disparities raised in our discussion. At least three types of initiatives to remedy information-sharing disparities seem promising: efforts to boost collective confidence (in people's understanding of health and science and, in turn, in their ability to start and engage conversations); efforts to meet people where they are by framing information in ways that resonate with audiences' everyday lives; and efforts to build community infrastructure by providing usable and convenient forums for neighbors and people with similar interests to share with one another. None of these three paths necessarily offers a quick fix. Each requires an orientation toward long-term planning and engagement with communities rather than short-term attempts simply to spread a particular message on a one-time basis.

Consequently, what we face is the short-term reality that peer-to-peer communication is not a guaranteed panacea and a long-term need for planning and investment to build and better understand the interpersonal networks in which people live their daily lives, particularly people whom we can classify as disadvantaged historically. Such tasks should begin now if we are to assist tomorrow's science and health communication personnel in succeeding with future promotion and education strategies. Community building, such as ensuring there are places where neighbors can express themselves and get to know each other, may not be an immediately popular investment given the lack of obvious short-term outcomes. Moreover, taking the extra step to frame stories and presentations in ways that resonate with everyday conversation also may seem like a waste to staff who worry more about scientific accuracy than pleasing audiences. Nonetheless, investments now in our abilities to connect with one another ultimately could offer relatively cost-effective, sustainable opportunities to promote information equality in key areas such as health and science by ensuring that we avoid the types of viral marketing and peer-to-peer campaign pitfalls outlined in this book.

Taking these extra steps now also will sow seeds for collective enrichment by increasing the sheer number of voices that contribute ideas to various debates, which is no small benefit given that 21st-century challenges posed by global disease and environmental changes promise to demand widespread sharing of whatever creativity humanity can muster. By acknowledging and addressing the reality of existing disparities between people and between communities in information sharing, we can work toward a future in which more people can participate in (and benefit from) ongoing dialogues, which in turn may help to craft healthier communities and even a healthier planet.

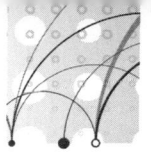

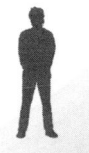

References

Chapter 1 References

1. Beaujon A. Despite media coverage, 45% of Americans don't know what Supreme Court ruled on health care. Poynter.org [Internet]. 2012 Jul 3 [cited 2012 Jul 3]. Available from: http://www.poynter.org/latest-news/mediawire/179785/despite-media-coverage-one-third-of-americans-dont-know-what-supreme-court-ruled-on-health-care

2. Politi D. Scientists find what looks like God particle. Slate [Internet]. 2012 Jul 4 [cited 2013 Mar 22]. Available from: http://slatest.slate.com/posts/2012/07/04/higgs_boson_cern_scientists_discover_what_looks_like_god_particle.html.

3. Gleick J. The information: a history, a theory, a flood. New York: Pantheon; 2011. 544 p.

4. Miller JD. Public understanding of, and attitudes toward, scientific research: what we know and what we need to know. Public Underst Sci. 2004;13:273-94.

5. Berkman ND, Davis TC, McCormack L. Health literacy: what is it? J Health Commun. 2010;15 Suppl 2:9-19.

6. McCormack L, Bann C, Uhrig J, Berkman N, Rudd R. Health insurance literacy of older adults. J Consumer Aff. 2009;43(2):223-48.

7. Severson K. Digital age is slow to arrive in rural America. New York Times. 2011 Feb 18. Sect. A:1.

8. Kontos EZ, Emmons KM, Puleo E, Viswanath K. Communication inequalities and public health implications of adult social networking site use in the United States. J Health Commun. 2010;15 Suppl 3:216-35.

Chapter 2 References

1. Taylor-Clark KA, Viswanath K, Blendon RJ. Communication inequalities during public health disasters: Katrina's wake. Health Commun. 2010 Apr;25(3):221-9.

2. Salathé M, Khandelwal S. Assessing vaccination sentiments with online social media: implications for infectious disease dynamics and control. PLoS Comput Biol. 2011 Oct;7(10):e1002199.

3. Tichenor PJ, Donohue GA, Olien CN. Mass media flow and differential growth in knowledge. Public Opin Q. 1970;34(2):159-70.

4. Viswanath K, Finnegan JR. The knowledge gap hypothesis: twenty-five years later. In: Burleson B, editor. Communication yearbook 19. Thousand Oaks, CA: Sage; 1996. p. 187-227.

5. Viswanath K, Breen N, Meissner H, Moser RP, Hesse B, Steele WR, Rakowski W. Cancer knowledge and disparities in the information age. J Health Commun. 2006;11 Suppl 1:1-17.

6. Gitlin T. Media unlimited: how the torrent of images and sounds overwhelms our lives. New York: Henry Holt and Company; 2003. p. 256.

7. Gleick J. The information: a history, a theory, a flood. New York: Pantheon; 2011. 544 p.

8. Kirchler E. Everyday life experiences at home: An interaction diary approach to assess marital relationships. J Fam Psychol. 1989;2:311-36.

9. Piselli, F. Communities, places, and social networks. Am Behav Sci. 2007;50(7):867-78.

10. Starbird K, Palen L. Pass it on?: Retweeting in mass emergency. Paper presented at: 7th International ISCRAM Conference; 2010 May; Seattle, WA.

11. Goldenberg J, Libai B, Muller E. Talk of the network: a complex system look at the underlying process of word-of-mouth. Marketing Lett. 2001;12:211-23.

12. Montgomery AL. Applying quantitative marketing techniques to the Internet. Interfaces. 2001;31(2):90-108.

13. Phelps JE, Lewis R, Mobilio L, Perry D, Raman N. Viral marketing or electronic word-of-mouth advertising: examining consumer responses and motivations to pass along email. J Advertising Res. 2004;44(4):333-48.

14. Rosen E. The anatomy of buzz: how to create word-of-mouth marketing. New York: Doubleday; 2002. 320 p.

15. Vilpponen A, Winter S, Sundqvist S. Electronic word-of-mouth in online environments: exploring referral network structure and adoption behavior. J Interactive Advertising. 2006;6(2):71-86.

16. De Bruyn A, Lilien GL. A multi-stage model of word-of-mouth influence through viral marketing. Int J Res Marketing. 2008;25:151-63.

17. Mohammed S. Personal communication networks and the effects of an entertainment-education radio soap opera in Tanzania. J Health Commun. 2001 Apr-Jun;6(2):137-54.

18. Gladwell M. The tipping point: how little things can make a big difference. New York: Little, Brown and Company; 2000. 288 p.

19. Lomas J, Enkin M, Anderson GM, Hannah WJ, Vayda E, Singer J. Opinion leaders vs audit and feedback to implement practice guidelines. Delivery after previous cesarean section. JAMA. 1991 May 1;265(17):2202-7.

20. L'Engle KL, Vahdat HL, Ndakidemi E, Lasway C, Zan T. Evaluating feasibility, reach and potential impact of a text message family planning information service in Tanzania. Contraception. 2013 Feb;87(2):251-6.

21. Tarde G. The laws of imitation. Parsons EC, translator. New York: H. Holt and Company; 1903. 404 p.

22. Katz E, Lazarsfeld PF. Personal influence. Glencoe, IL: Free Press; 1955. 434 p.

23. Dawkins R. The selfish gene. New York: Oxford University Press; 1976. 224 p.

24. Dorogovtsev SN, Mendes JF, Samukhin AN. Structure of growing networks with preferential linking. Phys Rev Lett. 2000 Nov 20;85(21):4633-6.

25. Newman ME. Clustering and preferential attachment in growing networks. Phys Rev E Stat Nonlin Soft Matter Phys. 2001 Aug;64(2 Pt 2):025102.

26. Barabási AL. Emergence of scaling in complex networks. In: Bornholdt S, Schuster HG, editors. Handbook of graph networks. Weinheim (Germany): Wiley-VCH; 2003. p. 69-84.

27. Himelboim I. Reply distribution in online discussions: a comparative network analysis of political and health newsgroups. J Comput-Mediated Commun. 2008;14:156-77.

28. Newman MEJ. The structure and function of complex networks. SIAM Rev. 2003;45(2):167-256.

29. Whitehead M. The concepts and principles of equity and health. Int J Health Serv. 1992;22(3):429-45.

30. Balarajan Y, Selvaraj S, Subramanian SV. Health care and equity in India. Lancet. 2011 Feb 5;377(9764):505-15.

31. Braveman P, Gruskin S. Defining equity in health. J Epidemiol Community Health. 2003 Apr;57(4):254-8.

32. Braveman P. Health disparities and health equity: concepts and measurement. Annu Rev Public Health. 2006;27:167-94.

33. Vivier PM, Hauptman M, Weitzen SH, Bell S, Quilliam DN, Logan JR. The important health impact of where a child lives: neighborhood characteristics and the burden of lead poisoning. Matern Child Health J. 2011 Nov;15(8):1195-202.

34. Watson B, Smithson-Stanley L, Riffe D, Ogilvie E. Mass media and perceived and objective environmental risk: race and place of residence. Howard J Commun. 2013 Apr;24:134-53.

Chapter 3 References

1. Castells M. The rise of the network society. 2nd ed. Oxford, UK: Wiley-Blackwell Publishing; 2000. 594 p.

2. Bobashev GV, Anthony JC. Clusters of marijuana use in the United States. Am J Epidemiol. 1998 Dec 15;148(12):1168-74.

3. Christakis NA, Fowler JH. Connected: the surprising power of our social networks and how they shape our lives. New York: Little, Brown and Company; 2009. 368 p.

4. Granovetter MS. The strength of weak ties. Am J Sociol. 1973;78(6): 1360-80.

5. Brown JJ, Reingen PH. Social ties and word-of-mouth referral behavior. J Consumer Res. 1987;14:350-62.

6. Moody J, White DR. Structural cohesion and embeddedness: A hierarchical concept of social groups. Am Sociol Rev. 2003;68(1):103-27.

7. Barabási AL. Emergence of scaling in complex networks. In: Bornholdt S, Schuster HG, editors. Handbook of graph networks. Weinheim (Germany): Wiley-VCH, 2003. p. 69-84.

8. Himelboim I. Reply distribution in online discussions: a comparative network analysis of political and health newsgroups. J Comput-Mediated Commun. 2008;14:156-77.

9. Southwell BG, Yzer MC. The roles of interpersonal communication in mass media campaigns. In: Beck C, editor. Communication yearbook 31. New York: Lawrence Erlbaum Associates; 2007. p. 420-62.

10. Cappella JN. Interpersonal communication: definitions and fundamental questions. In: Berger CR, Chaffee SH, editors. Handbook of communication science. Newbury Park, CA: Sage; 1987. p. 184-238.

11. Watzlawick P, Bavelas JHB, Jackson DD. Pragmatics of human communication: a study of interactional patterns, pathologies, and paradoxes. New York: Norton; 1967. 296 p.

12. Knapp ML, Daly JA, editors. Handbook of interpersonal communication. 2nd ed. Thousand Oaks, CA: Sage; 2002. 848 p.

13. Berger CR. Goals and knowledge structures in social interaction. In: Knapp ML, Daly JA, editors. Handbook of interpersonal communication. 3rd ed. Thousand Oaks, CA: Sage; 2002. p. 181-212.

14. Daly JA. Personality and interpersonal communication. In: Knapp ML, Daly JA, editors. Handbook of interpersonal communication. 3rd ed. Thousand Oaks, CA: Sage; 2002. p. 133-80.

15. Dillard JP, Anderson JW, Knobloch LK. Interpersonal influence. In: Knapp ML, Daly JA, editors. Handbook of interpersonal communication. 3rd ed. Thousand Oaks, CA: Sage; 2002. p. 423-74.

16. Poole MS, McPhee RD, Canary DJ, Morr MC. Hypothesis testing and modeling perspectives on inquiry. In: Knapp ML, Daly JA, editors. Handbook of interpersonal communication. 3rd ed. Thousand Oaks, CA: Sage; 2002. p. 23-72.

17. Walther JB, Parks MR. Cues filtered out, cues filtered in: computer-mediated communication and relationships. In: Knapp ML, Daly JA, editors. Handbook of interpersonal communication. 3rd ed. Thousand Oaks, CA: Sage; 2002. p. 529-63.

18. Roloff ME, Anastasiou L. Interpersonal communication research: an overview. In: Gudykunst WB, editor. Communication yearbook 24. Thousand Oaks, CA: Sage; 2001. p. 51-70.

19. Berger CR. Interpersonal communication: theoretical perspectives, future prospects. J Commun. 2005;55:415-47.

20. Starbird K, Palen L. Pass it on?: Retweeting in mass emergency. Paper presented at: 7th International ISCRAM Conference; 2010 May; Seattle, WA.

21. Knapp ML, Daly JA, Albada KF, Miller GR. Background and current trends in the study of interpersonal communication. In: Knapp ML, Daly JA, editors. Handbook of interpersonal communication. 3rd ed. Thousand Oaks, CA: Sage; 2002. p. 3-20.

22. Duffy B, Smith K, Terhanian G, Bremer J. Comparing data from online and face-to-face surveys. Int J Market Res. 2005;47:615-39.

23. Matsuba MK. Searching for self and relationships online. Cyber-Psychol Behav. 2006;9:275-84.

24. Price V, Nir L, Cappella JN. Normative and informational influences in online political discussions. Commun Theory. 2006;16:47-74.

25. Herring S. Interactional coherence in CMC. J Comput-Mediated Commun. 1999;4(4). Available from: http://jcmc.indiana.edu/vol4/issue4/herring.html.

26. Baym NK, Zhang YB, Lin MC. Social interactions across media: interpersonal communication on the Internet, telephone, and face-to-face. New Media Soc. 2004;6:299-318.

27. Papacharissi Z. The real-virtual dichotomy in online interaction: new media uses and consequences revisited. In: Kalbfleisch PJ, editor. Communication yearbook 29. Mahwah, NJ: Lawrence Erlbaum Associates; 2005. p. 215-37.

28. Fishbein M, Ajzen I. Predicting and changing behavior: the reasoned action approach. New York: Psychology Press; 2010. 538 p.

29. Carr N. The shallows: what the Internet is doing to our brains. New York: W. W. Norton & Company; 2011. 280 p.

30. Lee KM. Presence, explicated. Commun Theory. 2004;14(1):27-50.

31. Cortese J, Seo M. The role of social presence in opinion expression during FtF and CMC discussions. Commun Res Rep. 2012;29(1):44-53.

Chapter 4 References

1. Banerjee N. The science behind Hurricane Sandy: a confluence of trouble. Los Angeles Times [Internet]. 2012 Oct 29 [cited 22 Mar 2013]. Available from: http://articles.latimes.com/2012/oct/29/nation/la-na-sandy-science-20121030.

2. Diez Roux AV. Conceptual approaches to the study of health disparities. Annu Rev Public Health. 2012 Apr;33:41-58.

3. Miller JD. Public understanding of, and attitudes toward, scientific research: what we know and what we need to know. Public Understanding Sci. 2004;13:273-94.

4. Oelschlegel S, Earl M, Taylor M, Muenchen RA. Health information disparities? determining the relationship between age, poverty, and rate of calls to a consumer and patient health information service. J Med Libr Assoc. 2009 Jul;97(3):225-7.

5. Nisbet MC, Scheufele DA. What's next for science communication? Promising directions and lingering distractions. Am J Botany. 2009; 96(10):1767-78.

6. Katz E, Lazarsfeld PF. Personal influence. Glencoe, IL: Free Press; 1955. 434 p.

7. Rogers EM. Diffusion of innovations. 1st ed. New York: The Free Press; 1962. 367 p.

8. Kim S, Southwell BG, Slater JS. Socioeconomic disparities in peer referral and information sharing about mammography. Paper presented at: International Communication Association Annual Conference; 2011 May; Boston, MA.

9. Mohammed S. Personal communication networks and the effects of an entertainment-education radio soap opera in Tanzania. J Health Commun. 2001 Apr-Jun;6(2):137-54.

10. Southwell BG, Gilkerson ND, Depue JB, Friedenberg LM. The conversation gap hypothesis: education and disparity in talk about media content. Paper presented at: National Communication Association Annual Conference; 2010 November; San Francisco, CA.

11. Seeman M, Evans JW. Alienation and learning in a hospital setting. Am Sociol Rev. 1962;27:772-82.

12. Hass A, Sherman MA. Conversational topic as a function of role and gender. Psychol Rep. 1982;51:453-4.

13. Sehulster JR. Things we talk about, how frequently, and to whom: frequency of topics in everyday conversation as a function of gender, age, and marital status. Am J Psychol. 2006;119:407-32.

14. Wagner W. Vernacular science knowledge: its role in everyday life communication. Public Understanding Sci. 2007;16:7-22.

15. Southwell BG, Torres A. Connecting interpersonal and mass communication: science news exposure, perceived ability to understand science, and conversation. Commun Monogr. 2006;73(3):334-50.

16. Southwell B, Murphy J, DeWaters J, LeBaron P. Energy information sharing in social networks: the roles of objective knowledge and perceived understanding. Paper presented at: Behavior, Energy, & Climate Change Conference; 2012 November; Sacramento, CA.

17. Weimann G. The influentials: back to the concept of opinion leaders. Public Opin Q. 1991;55:267-79.

18. McCroskey JC. Oral communication apprehension: a summary of recent theory and research. Hum Commun Res. 1977;4:78-96.

19. McCroskey JC, Richmond VP. Community size as a predictor of development of communication apprehension: replication and extension. Commun Education. 1978;27:212-9.

20. McCroskey JC, Richmond VP. Communication apprehension and shyness: conceptual and operational distinctions. Cent States Speech J. 1982;33:458-68.

21. Sorensen G, McCroskey JC. The prediction of interaction behavior in small groups: zero history vs. intact groups. Commun Monogr. 1977;44:73-80.

22. Zuckerman M. Behavioral expressions and biosocial bases of sensation seeking. Cambridge, UK: Cambridge University Press; 1994. 480 p.

23. Roberti JW. A review of behavioral and biological correlates of sensation seeking. J Res Pers. 2004;38:256-79.

24. Stephenson MT, Morgan SE, Lorch EP, Palmgreen P, Donohew L, Hoyle RH. Predictors of exposure from an antimarijuana media campaign: outcome research assessing sensation seeking targeting. Health Commun. 2002;14(1):23-43.

25. Stephenson MT, Southwell BG. Sensation seeking, the activation model, and mass media health campaigns: current findings and future directions for cancer communication. J Commun. 2006;56:s38-s56.

26. Zuckerman M, Kuhlman S. Personality and risk-taking: common biosocial factors. J Pers. 2000;68:999-1029.

27. Strauman TJ, Wilson WA. Individual differences in approach and avoidance. In: Hoyle, RH, editor. Handbook of personality and self-regulation [Internet]. Oxford, UK: Wiley-Blackwell; 2010. Chapter 20. doi: 10.1002/9781444318111.ch20.

28. Lang A, Shin M, Lee S. Sensation seeking, motivation, and substance use: a dual system approach. Media Psychol. 2005;7:1-29.

29. Netter P, Rammsayer TH. Reactivity to dopaminergic drugs and aggression related to personality traits. Pers Individual Differences. 1991;12:1009-17.

30. Rammsayer TH. Extraversion and the dopamine hypothesis. In: Stelmack RM, editor. On the psychobiology of personality: essays in honor of Marvin Zuckerman. Ottawa, Canada: Elsevier; 2004. p. 409-27.

31. Donohew L, Bardo MT, Zimmerman RS. Personality and risky behavior: Communication and prevention. In: Stelmack RM, editor. On the psychobiology of personality: essays in honor of Marvin Zuckerman. Ottawa, Canada: Elsevier; 2004. p. 223-45.

32. Martin BA, Sherrard MJ, Wentzel D. The role of sensation seeking and need for cognition on Web-site evaluations: a resource matching perspective. Psychol Marketing. 2005;22(2):109-26.

33. Bardo MT, Donohew RL, Harrington NG. Psychobiology of novelty seeking and drug seeking behavior. Behav Brain Res. 1996 May;77(1-2):23-43.

34. Zuckerman M. The psychobiological model for impulsive unsocialized sensation seeking: a comparative approach. Neuropsychobiology. 1996;34(3):125-9.

35. Zuckerman M, Persky H, Link KE. Experimental and subject factors determining responses to sensory deprivation, social isolation, and confinement. J Abnorm Psychol. 1968 Jun;73(3):183-94.

36. Franken RE, Gibson KJ, Mohan P. Sensation seeking and disclosure to close and casual friends. Pers Individual Differences. 1990;11(8):829-32.

37. Zuckerman M, Link K. Construct validity for the sensation-seeking scale. J Consult Clin Psychol. 1968 Aug;32(4):420-6.

38. David C, Cappella JN, Fishbein M. The social diffusion of influence among adolescents: Group interaction in a chat room environment about anti-drug advertisements. Commun Theory. 2006;16:118-40.

39. Hwang Y, Southwell BG. Can a personality trait predict talk about science? Sensation seeking as a science communication targeting variable. Sci Commun. 2007;29(2):198-216.

Chapter 5 References

1. Katz E, Lazarsfeld PF. Personal influence. Glencoe, IL: Free Press; 1955. 434 p.

2. Gladwell M. The tipping point: how little things can make a big difference. New York: Little, Brown and Company; 2000. 288 p.

3. Katz E. The two-step flow of communication: an up-to-date report on an hypothesis. Public Opin Q. 1957;21(1):61-78.

4. Kadushin C. Personal influence: a radical theory of action. Ann Am Acad Pol Soc Sci. 2006;608:270-81.

5. Snyder M, Omoto AM. Volunteerism: social issues perspectives and social policy implications. Soc Issues Policy Rev. 2008;2(1):1-36.

6. Watts DJ. Challenging the influentials hypothesis. In: Carl WJ, editor. Measuring word of mouth: volume 3. Chicago, IL: Word of Mouth Marketing Association; 2007. p. 201-11.

7. Dodds PS, Watts DJ. Universal behavior in a generalized model of contagion. Phys Rev Lett. 2004 May 28;92(21):218701.

8. Dodds PS, Watts DJ. A generalized model of social and biological contagion. J Theor Biol. 2005 Feb 21;232(4):587-604.

9. Morgan SE. The intersection of conversation, cognitions, and campaigns: the social representation of organ donation. Commun Theory. 2009;19(1):29-48.

10. Sohn D. Disentangling the effects of social network density on electronic word-of-mouth (eWOM) intention. J Comput-Mediated Commun. 2009;14:352-67.

11. Lee HM. Social representations, social networks, and public relations effects: the consequences of exposure to sided media content in different interpersonal settings [dissertation]. [Minneapolis]: University of Minnesota; 2011. 198 p.

12. Burt RS. Social contagion and innovation: Cohesion versus structural equivalence. Am J Sociol. 1987;92(6):1287-335.

13. Coleman JS, Katz E, Menzel H. Medical innovation. New York: Bobbs-Merrill; 1966. 246 p.

14. Kawachi I, Kennedy BP, Lochner K, Prothrow-Stith D. Social capital, income inequality, and mortality. Am J Public Health. 1997 Sep;87(9):1491-8.

15. Putnam R. Bowling alone: the collapse and revival of American community. New York: Simon & Schuster; 2000. 546 p.

16. Husaini BA, Sherkat DE, Levine R, Bragg R, Van CA, Emerson JS, Mentes CM. The effect of a church-based breast cancer screening education program on mammography rates among African-American women. J Natl Med Assoc. 2002 Feb;94(2):100-6.

17. Frank KA, Zhao Y, Borman K. Social capital and the diffusion of innovations within organizations: the case of computer technology in schools. Sociol Educ. 2004;77(2):148-71.

18. Derose KP. Do bonding, bridging, and linking social capital affect preventable hospitalizations? Health Serv Res. 2008 Oct;43(5 Pt 1):1520-41.

19. Bourdieu P. The forms of capital. In: J. Richardson, editor. Handbook of theory and research for the sociology of education. New York: Greenwood; 1986. p. 241-58.

20. Coleman JS. Social capital in the creation of human capital. Am J Sociol. 1988;94:s95-s120.

21. Coleman JS. Foundations of social theory. Cambridge, MA: Harvard University Press; 1990. 1014 p.

22. Cummins S, Macintyre S, Davidson S, Ellaway A. Measuring neighbourhood social and material context: generation and interpretation of ecological data from routine and non-routine sources. Health Place. 2005 Sep;11(3):249-60.

23. Beaudoin CE. Bonding and bridging neighborliness: an individual-level study in the context of health. Soc Sci Med. 2009 Jun;68(12):2129-36.

24. Curley AM. Draining or gaining? The social networks of public housing in Boston. J Soc Personal Relationships. 2009;26(2-3):227-47.

25. Portes A. Social capital: its origins and applications in modern sociology. Ann Rev Sociol. 1998;24:1-24.

26. Carpiano RM. Toward a neighborhood resource-based theory of social capital for health: can Bourdieu and sociology help? Soc Sci Med. 2006 Jan;62(1):165-75.

27. Stephens C. Social capital in its place: using social theory to understand social capital and inequalities in health. Soc Sci Med. 2008 Mar;66(5):1174-84.

28. Mulvaney-Day NE, Alegría M, Sribney W. Social cohesion, social support, and health among Latinos in the United States. Soc Sci Med. 2007 Jan; 64(2):477-95.

29. Southwell BG, Slater JS, Rothman AJ, Friedenberg LM, Allison TR, Nelson CL. The availability of community ties predicts likelihood of peer referral for mammography: geographic constraints on viral marketing. Soc Sci Med. 2010 Nov;71(9):1627-35.

30. Viswanath K, Kosicki GM, Fredin ES, Park E. Local community ties, community-boundedness, and local public affairs knowledge gaps. Commun Res. 2000;27(1):27-50.

31. Lapinski MK, Rimal RN. An explication of social norms. Commun Theory. 2005;15:127-47.

32. Phelps JE, Lewis R, Mobilio L, Perry D, Raman N. Viral marketing or electronic word-of-mouth advertising: examining consumer responses and motivations to pass along email. J Advertising Res. 2004;44(4):333-48.

33. Sundaram DS, Mitra K, Webster C. Word-of-mouth communications: a motivational analysis. In: Alba JW, Hutchinson JW, editors. Advances in consumer research: volume 25. Chicago: Association for Consumer Research; 1998. p. 527-31.

34. Hogg MA. A social identity theory of leadership. Pers Soc Psychol Rev. 2001;5:184-200.

35. Hogg MA, Reid SA. Social identity, self-categorization, and the communication of group norms. Commun Theory. 2006;16:7-30.

36. van Knippenberg D, van Knippenberg B, De Cremer D, Hogg MA. Leadership, self, and identity: a review and research agenda. Leadership Q. 2004;15:825-56.

37. Brabham DC. Motivations for participation in a crowdsourcing application to improve public engagement in transit planning. J Appl Commun Res. 2012;40(3):307-28.

38. Oishi S, Rothman AJ, Snyder M, Su J, Zehm K, Hertel AW, Gonzales MH, Sherman GD. The socioecological model of procommunity action: the benefits of residential stability. J Pers Soc Psychol. 2007 Nov;93(5):831-44.

39. Kasarda JD, Janowitz M. Community attachment in mass society. Am Sociol Rev. 1974;39:328-39.

40. Schieman S. Residential stability and the social impact of neighborhood disadvantage: a study of gender- and race-contingent effects. Soc Forces. 2005;83(3):1031-64.

41. Borgatti SP, Cross R. A relational view of information seeking and learning in social networks. Manage Sci. 2003;49(4):432-45.

42. Brennan EM. Changing smoking behaviour: the contribution of interpersonal communication to mass media campaign effects [dissertation]. [Melbourne, Australia]: University of Melbourne; 2012. 429 p.

43. Negin J, Wariero J, Mutuo P, Jan S, Pronyk P. Feasibility, acceptability and cost of home-based HIV testing in rural Kenya. Trop Med Int Health. 2009 Aug;14(8):849-55.

44. Freeman B, Chapman S. Gone viral? Heard the buzz? A guide for public health practitioners and researchers on how Web 2.0 can subvert advertising restrictions and spread health information. J Epidemiol Community Health. 2008 Sep;62(9):778-82.

45. Nepal V, Banerjee D, Perry M, Scott D. Disaster preparedness of linguistically isolated populations: practical issues for planners. Health Promot Pract. 2012 Mar;13(2):265-71.

46. Fant L. Cultural mismatch in conversations: Spanish and Scandinavian communicative behaviour in negotiations settings. Hermes J Linguistics. 1989;3:247-65.

47. Realo A, Goodwin R. Family-related allocentrism and HIV risk behavior in Central and Eastern Europe. J Cross-Cultural Psychol. 2003;34(6):690-701.

48. Morse DS, Paldi Y, Egbarya SS, Clark CJ. "An effect that is deeper than beating": family violence in Jordanian women. Fam Syst Health. 2012 Mar;30(1):19-31.

49. Davis RE, Resnicow K, Couper MP. Survey response styles, acculturation, and culture among a sample of Mexican American adults. J Cross-Cultural Psychol. 2011;42(7):1219-36.

50. Schumann JH, Wangenheim Fv, Stringfellow A, Yang Z, Blazevic V, Praxmarer, S. Cross-cultural differences in the effect of received word-of-mouth referral in relational service exchange. J Int Marketing. 2010;18(3):62-80.

51. Ren XS, Amick B 3rd, Zhou L, Gandek B. Translation and psychometric evaluation of a Chinese version of the SF-36 Health Survey in the United States. J Clin Epidemiol. 1998 Nov;51(11):1129-38.

Chapter 6 References

1. Friedenberg LM, Wang Y, Choi TCK, Southwell BG, Lazovich D, Forster J. Family communication constraints as health intervention challenge: Parent-child conversation about indoor tanning. Paper presented at: American Public Health Association Annual Meeting. 2009 Nov. Philadelphia, PA.

2. Wright CR. Mass communication: a sociological perspective. New York: McGraw-Hill; 1986. 236 p.

3. Himelboim I. Reply distribution in online discussions: a comparative network analysis of political and health newsgroups. J Comput-Mediated Commun. 2008;14:156-77.

4. Watts DJ. Challenging the influentials hypothesis. In: Carl WJ, editor. Measuring word of mouth: volume 3. Chicago: Word of Mouth Marketing Association; 2007. p. 201-11.

5. Morgan SE. The intersection of conversation, cognitions, and campaigns: the social representation of organ donation. Commun Theory 2009;19(1):29-40.

6. Moscovici S. The history and actuality of social representations. In: Flick U, editor. The psychology of the social. Cambridge: Cambridge University Press; 1998. p. 209-47.

7. Blackmore S. The meme machine. New York: Oxford University Press; 1999. 288 p.

8. Dawkins R. The selfish gene. New York: Oxford University Press; 1976. 224 p.

9. Hoeken H, Swanepoel P, Saal E, Jansen C. Using message form to stimulate conversations: the case of tropes. Commun Theory. 2009;19(1):49-65.

10. Kennedy GA. Aristotle, on rhetoric: a theory of civic discourse. New York: Oxford University Press; 1991. 335 p.

11. Tanaka, K. The pun in advertising. Lingua. 1992;87:91-102.

12. Tanaka, K. Advertising language: a pragmatic approach to advertisements in Britain and Japan. London: Routledge; 1994. 168 p.

13. Southwell BG, Torres A. Connecting interpersonal and mass communication: science news exposure, perceived ability to understand science, and conversation. Commun Monogr. 2006;73(3):334-50.

14. Dunlop SM, Wakefield M, Kashima Y. The contribution of antismoking advertising to quitting: intra- and interpersonal processes. J Health Commun. 2008 Apr-May;13(3):250-66.

15. Hafstad A, Aaro LE. Activating interpersonal influence through provocative appeals: evaluation of a mass media-based antismoking campaign targeting adolescents. Health Commun. 1997;9:253-72.

16. Dunlop SM, Kashima Y, Wakefield M. Predictors and consequences of conversations about health promoting media messages. Commun Monogr. 2010;77(4):518-39.

17. Brennan EM. Changing smoking behaviour: the contribution of interpersonal communication to mass media campaign effects [dissertation]. [Melbourne, Australia]: University of Melbourne; 2012. 429 p.

18. Berger J. Arousal increases social transmission of information. Psychol Sci. 2011;22(7):891-3.

19. Berger J, Milkman KL. What makes online content viral? J Marketing Res. 2012;49(2):192-205.

20. Schriner M. Where is the revolution? Health news on the Internet: online user preferences and their contrasts with prevalence of private-sector originating sources [dissertation]. [Minneapolis]: University of Minnesota; 2011. 126 p.

21. Rimé B, Mesquita B, Philippot P, Boca S. Beyond the emotional event: six studies on the social sharing of emotion. Cogn Emotion. 1991;5:435-65.

22. Mendolia M, Kleck RE. Effects of talking about a stressful event on arousal: does what we talk about make a difference? J Pers Soc Psychol. 1993:64:283-92.

23. Allport GW, Postman LJ. The psychology of rumor. New York: Holt, Rinehart & Winston; 1947. 247 p.

24. Weeks BE, Friedenberg LM, Southwell BG, Slater JS. Behavioral consequences of conflict-oriented health news coverage: the 2009 mammography guideline controversy and online information seeking. Health Commun. 2012;27(2):158-66.

25. Nabi RL. A cognitive-functional model for the effects of discrete negative emotions on information processing, attitude change, and recall. Commun Theory. 1999;9(3):292-320.

26. Dillard JP, Nabi R. The persuasive influence of emotion in cancer prevention and detection messages. J Commun. 2006;56:S123-39.

27. Peters K, Kashima Y, Clark A. Talking about others: emotionality and the dissemination of social information. European J Soc Psychol. 2009;39(2):207-22.

28. Hwang Y, Southwell BG. Science TV news exposure predicts science beliefs: real world effects among a national sample. Commun Res. 2009;36(5):724-42.

29. Southwell BG, Slater JS, Nelson CL, Rothman AJ. Does it pay to pay people to share information? Using financial incentives to promote peer referral for mammography among the underinsured. Am J Health Promot. 2012 Jul-Aug;26(6):348-51.

Chapter 7 References

1. Southwell BG, Yzer MC. When (and why) interpersonal talk matters for campaigns. Commun Theory. 2009;19(1):1-8.

2. Tichenor PJ, Donohue GA, Olien CN. Mass media flow and differential growth in knowledge. Public Opin Q. 1970;34(2):159-70.

3. van den Putte B, Yzer M, Southwell BG, de Bruijn GJ, Willemsen MC. Interpersonal communication as an indirect pathway for the effect of antismoking media content on smoking cessation. J Health Commun. 2011 May;16(5):470-85.

4. Lenart S. Shaping political attitudes: the impact of interpersonal communication and mass media. Thousand Oaks, CA: Sage; 1994. 150 p.

5. Scheufele DA. Examining differential gains from mass media and their implication for participatory behavior. Commun Res. 2002;29:46-65.

6. Eveland WP. The effect of political discussion in producing informed citizens: the roles of information, motivation, and elaboration. Political Commun. 2004;21:177-93.

7. Dickinson C, Givon T. Memory and conversation: toward an experimental paradigm. In: Givon T, editor. Conversation: cognitive, communicative, and social perspectives. Amsterdam, Netherlands: John Benjamins; 1997. p. 91-132.

8. Edwards D, Middleton D. Conversation and remembering: Bartlett revisited. Appl Cogn Psychol. 1987;1:77-92.

9. Southwell BG. Between messages and people: a multilevel model of memory for television content. Commun Res. 2005;32(1):112-40.

10. Bower GH. A brief history of memory research. In: Tulving E, Craik FIM, editors. The Oxford handbook of memory. New York: Oxford University Press; 2000. p. 3-32.

11. Fuster JM. Memory in the cerebral cortex: an empirical approach to neural networks in the human and nonhuman primate. Cambridge, MA: MIT Press; 1999. 372 p.

12. Anderson JR. The architecture of cognition. Cambridge, MA: Harvard University Press; 1983. 345 p.

13. Anderson JR. Cognitive psychology and its implications. 3rd ed. New York: W. H. Freeman; 1990. 519 p.

14. Wirtz JG. Mass media campaigns and conversation: testing short-term and long-term priming effects of topic-related conversation on conversational participants [dissertation]. [Minneapolis]: University of Minnesota; 2009. 246 p.

15. Robinson JP, Davis DK. Television news and the informed public: an information-processing approach. J Commun. 1990;40(3):106-19.

16. Southwell BG. Interpersonal influence: conversation sparks memory for science-related media content. Paper presented at: Association for Education in Journalism and Mass Communication annual convention; 2005 Aug; San Antonio, TX.

17. van den Putte B, Yzer M, Southwell B. Health campaign exposure and interpersonal communication: moderating and mediating effects. Health Psychol Rev. 2007;1 Suppl 1:214.

18. Carr N. The shallows: what the Internet is doing to our brains. New York: W. W. Norton & Company; 2011. 280 p

19. Yzer M, Southwell B, Rothman A. Talk with others and norm perceptions as distinct influences on marijuana use. Ann Behav Med. 2012;43 Suppl:s215.

20. Hornik R, Yanovitzky I. Using theory to design evaluations of communication campaigns: the case of the National Youth Anti-Drug Media Campaign. Commun Theory. 2003;13:204-24.

21. Valente TW, Saba WP. Mass media and interpersonal influence in a reproductive health communication campaign in Bolivia. Commun Res. 1998;25:96-124.

22. Valente TW, Saba WP. Campaign exposure and interpersonal communication as factors in contraceptive use in Bolivia. J Health Commun. 2001 Oct-Dec;6(4):303-22.

23. Durkin S, Wakefield M. Maximising the impact of emotive anti-tobacco advertising: effects of interpersonal discussion and program placement. Soc Marketing Q. 2006;12(3):3-14.

24. David C, Cappella JN, Fishbein M. The social diffusion of influence among adolescents: group interaction in a chat room environment about anti-drug advertisements. Commun Theory. 2006;26:118-40.

25. Compton JA, Pfau M. Use of inoculation to foster resistance to credit card marketing targeting college students. J Appl Commun Res. 2004;32:343-64.

26. Compton J, Pfau M. Spreading inoculation: Inoculation, resistance to influence, and word-of-mouth communication. Commun Theory. 2009;19(1):9-28.

27. Beghin JC, Jensen HH. Farm policies and added sugars in US diets. Food Policy. 2008;33(6):480-8.

28. Koplan JP, Liverman CT, Kraak VI, editors. Preventing childhood obesity: health in the balance. Washington, DC: The National Academies Press; 2005. 436 p.

29. Richardson CR, Buis LR, Janney AW, Goodrich DE, Sen A, Hess ML, Mehari KS, Fortlage LA, Resnick PJ, Zikmund-Fisher BJ, Strecher VJ, Piette JD. An online community improves adherence in an Internet-mediated walking program. Part 1: results of a randomized controlled trial. J Med Internet Res. 2010 Dec 17;12(4):e71.

30. Moody J, White DR. Structural cohesion and embeddedness: a hierarchical concept of social groups. Am Sociol Rev. 2003;68(1):103-27.

Chapter 8 References

1. Sen A. Inequality reexamined. New York: Oxford University Press; 2003. doi: 10.1093/0198289286.001.0001

2. Lippmann W. Public opinion. New York: Macmillan; 1922. 427 p.

3. Lippmann W. The phantom public. New York: Macmillan; 1925. 205 p.

4. Nisbet MC, Scheufele DA. What's next for science communication? Promising directions and lingering distractions. Am J Botany. 2009;96(10):1767-78.

5. Brossard D, Nisbet MC. Deference to scientific authority among a low information public: understanding American views about agricultural biotechnology. Int J Public Opin Res. 2007;19:24-52.

6. Southwell BG, Torres A. Connecting interpersonal and mass communication: science news exposure, perceived ability to understand science, and conversation. Commun Monogr. 2006;73(3):334-50.

7. Southwell B, Murphy J, DeWaters J, LeBaron P. Energy information sharing in social networks: the roles of objective knowledge and perceived understanding. Paper presented at: Behavior, Energy, & Climate Change Conference; 2012 Nov; Sacramento, CA.

8. Hilgartner S. The dominant view of popularization: conceptual problems, political uses. Soc Stud Sci. 1990;20:519-39.

9. Logan RA. Popularization versus secularization: media coverage of health. In: Wilkin L, Patterson P. Risky business: communicating issues of science, risk, and public policy. New York, NY: Greenwood Press; 1991. p. 43-59.

10. Gurak LJ, Lannon JM. A concise guide to technical communication. 4th ed. New York, NY: Pearson Longman; 2004. 352 p.

11. Nisbet MC, Scheufele DA. The future of public engagement. Scientist. 2007 Oct;39-44.

12. Payton FC, Kiwanuka-Tondo J, Kvasny L. Black female voices: designing an HIV information artifact. Paper presented at: 4th International Conference on the Applied Human Factors and Ergonomics; 2012 Jul; San Francisco, CA.

13. Horner JR. Conversation, social capital, and bureaucracy: talking about rights for the disabled in an online support group. Paper presented at: International Communication Association Annual Conference; 2001 May; Washington, DC.

14. Rupert DJ, Gard JC, Moultrie RR, Amoozegar JB, Aikin K, O'Donoghue A, Sullivan H. How Do online health communities influence medical treatment decisions? Examining patient and caregiver experiences. Paper presented at: American Public Health Association Annual Meeting; 2012 Nov; San Francisco, CA.

15. Gavin J, Rodham K, Poyer H. The presentation of "pro-anorexia" in online group interactions. Qual Health Res. 2008 Mar;18(3):325-33.

16. Nerlich B. "Climategate": paradoxical metaphors and political paralysis. Environ Values. 2010;19(4):419-42.

17. Frost JH, Massagli MP. Social uses of personal health information within PatientsLikeMe, an online patient community: what can happen when patients have access to one another's data. J Med Internet Res. 2008 May 27;10(3):e15.

18. Cobb NK, Graham AL, Abrams DB. Social network structure of a large online community for smoking cessation. Am J Public Health. 2010 Jul;100(7):1282-9.

19. Hampton KN. Internet use and the concentration of disadvantage: glocalization and the urban underclass. Am Behav Scientist. 2010;53(8):1111-32.

20. Severson K. Digital age is slow to arrive in rural America. New York Times. 2011 Feb 18. Sect. A:1.

21. Kontos EZ, Emmons KM, Puleo E, Viswanath K. Communication inequalities and public health implications of adult social networking site use in the United States. J Health Commun. 2010;15 Suppl 3:216-35.

22. White CM. Social media, crisis communication, and emergency management: leveraging web 2.0 technologies. Boca Raton, FL: CRC Press; 2012. 329 p.

About the Author

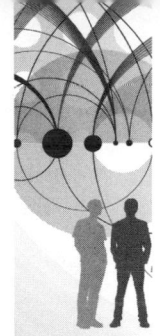

Brian G. Southwell, PhD, is a senior research scientist at RTI International, a nonprofit research institute headquartered in Research Triangle Park, North Carolina. He is also a faculty member at both the University of North Carolina at Chapel Hill and Duke University. At UNC, he holds appointments in the School of Journalism and Mass Communication and the Gillings School of Global Public Health. At Duke, he is affiliated with the Duke University Energy Initiative. Two principle foci of his research have been public understanding of science and the evaluation of large-scale mass media campaigns. His interest in social networks stems in part from his work on factors that moderate societal information flow and mass media effects.

Originally from upstate New York, Dr. Southwell holds degrees from the University of Virginia and the University of Pennsylvania. Following the completion of his doctorate, he served almost a decade at the University of Minnesota, where he was an associate professor and Director of Graduate Studies in the School of Journalism and Mass Communication, with an adjunct appointment in the School of Public Health. Dr. Southwell also has worked for a variety of nonprofit and government organizations, including the US Centers for Disease Control and Prevention in Atlanta, Georgia, as well as Ogilvy Public Relations in Washington, DC.

Dr. Southwell's research has been funded by the National Science Foundation, the National Institutes of Health, and other sources, and he has led a number of projects for agencies such as the US Food and Drug Administration. His published work has appeared in a wide variety of peer-reviewed journals such as *Social Science and Medicine* and *Communication Research* and in a number of books. Dr. Southwell also has served as editor for a number of publications, including work as senior editor for *Health Communication*, guest co-editor for *Communication Theory*, and member of the editorial boards of *Public Opinion Quarterly* and five other journals. His doctoral dissertation was recognized as a Dissertation of the Year jointly by the International Communication Association and the National Communication Association. In 2006, he was awarded the Arthur "Red" Motley Exemplary Teaching Award at the University of Minnesota. In 2011, he was recognized with the President's Award at RTI International. In 2012, Southwell and co-author Marco Yzer were awarded the Distinguished Article Award by the Health Communication division of the National Communication Association for their 2007 *Communication Yearbook* piece in recognition of its five-year impact.

Dr. Southwell lives with his family in Chapel Hill.

Index

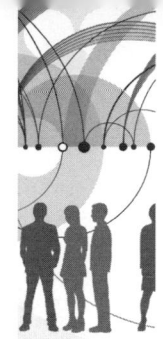

A

access to information: differences in, 7; equal, 94; to health information, 94–95, 102; via Internet, 102

advertising: anti-drug advertisements, 43, 83–84, 84–85, 86–87; anti-smoking advertisements, 58–59, 70–71; anti-tobacco advertisements, 26–27, 86; gross ratings points for, 85; memory of, 83–84, 84f; translation of advertisement exposure into memory, 83–84, 84f; word-of-mouth, 10–11

Affordable Care Act (Patient Protection and Affordable Care Act), 1, 2, 64–65

African Americans, 38, 61–62

alienation, 35–36

altruism, 54

American Institute of Physics, 73

anti-drug campaigns: advertisements, 43, 83–84, 84–85, 86–87; public service announcements, 86–87

anti-smoking campaigns: advertisements, 26–27, 58–59, 70–71, 86; mass media campaigns, 79; QuitNet, 101

anti-tobacco advertisements, 26–27

anticipatory elaboration, 79–80

argument resistance, 88–89

arousal, 20, 42, 71

attachment, preferential, 13

audience involvement, 82, 103–104

Australia, 61, 70–71, 86

B

BAS. *see* behavioral approach system

behavior, information-sharing, 17–29, 21f

behavioral approach system (BAS), 42

behavioral inhibition system (BIS), 42

bonding, social, 52, 55–56

boosting collective confidence, 97–98

boosting confidence, 72–74

bridging: community ties, 51–53, 54–56, 56–57, 99–103; strong ties, 20; weak ties, 18–19, 20, 52

bridging hubs, 32

Buffalo, New York, 38

C

capital, social, 51–53, 55–56

Carolina Donor Services, 27

Caucasians, 38

China, 61

Chinese, 61–62

Clean Energy Durham, 97–98

climate change, 34, 35

Climategate, 100–101

clustering, social, 18–19

cognitive salience, 81–85, 89

collective confidence, 97–98

commentary, 26–27

communication: online discussions, 19–20, 99–100; oral, 41; peer-to-peer, 105–106; viral, 10–11. *see also* conversation; talk

communication apprehension, 40–41

communication technology, 6, 102

communities: building, 99–103, 105–106; endurance of, 56; example, 56–57; factors that affect information sharing, 47–62; residential stability of, 56–57; variables that describe, 47

community building, 99–103, 105–106

community preparedness, 103

community ties: available, 51–53; building connections, 99–103; example, 56–57; and information sharing, 54–56; strong ties, 20; weak ties, 18–19, 20, 52

confidence boosting, 72–74, 97–98

congregation density, 57

connective technology, 102, 103

Note: Page numbers followed by *f* or *t* indicate figures or tables, respectively.

contextual understanding, 62
conversation: as behavioral phenomenon, 22; cultural differences in, 60; definition of, 22; as information-sharing behavior, 21*f*, 22–23; as interaction, 22; online chat, 24–25; online discussions, 19–20; partner availability and, 49; planned, 23; preparation for, 80; at Thanksgiving, 37. *see also* talk
conversation drivers, 70
conversation gaps, 8–10
conversational permissiveness, 58
cooptation, 21*f*, 26–27
credit card marketing: inoculation against, 88–89; vulnerability to, 88–89
crowdsourcing, 55
cultural differences, 48–49, 59–62
culture, 60–61

D

DBIS. *see* Discoveries and Breakthroughs Inside Science
denigration. *see* protest & denigration
density: congregation density, 57; of social networks, 49–50
designated market areas, 38
diffusion of information, 12–13
diffusion of memes, 68
Discoveries and Breakthroughs Inside Science (DBIS) project, 73
discussions online, 19–20, 99–100
dissemination of information, 93–94. *see also* information sharing
dopamine, 42
drug use: anti-drug campaigns, 43, 83–84, 84–85, 86–87; attitudes toward, 83–84; promoting prescription drugs, 59, 61–62

E

e-mailed stories, 64–65, 65*t*, 66*t*
early adopters, 32
education, 33, 34–36
elaboration, anticipatory, 79–80
ellipsis, rhetorical, 68–69
emergency management, 103
emotional response, 70–72
endorsement, overt, 21*f*, 25–26
energy information sharing, 39
engagement, 91
engineering, 44
environmental health, 34, 35
ethnic background, 38, 102

F

Facebook, 17, 21, 24, 25, 103
families, 58
familism, 61
family planning, 34
Federal Transit Administration, 55
financial incentives, 27, 74–75
Florida, 26–27
forwarding: e-mailed stories, 64–65, 65*t*, 66*t*; as information-sharing behavior, 21*f*, 24–25; of memes, 67–68; stories most likely to be forwarded, 67; of text messages, 56
fragile X advocacy groups, 100
fragile X syndrome online discussion forums, 99–100
framing of information, 7–8

G

Gangnam style, 12
Germany, 61
global warming, 35
"God particle" (Higgs Boson), 2–3
Google+, 17, 25
gregariousness, 40
gross ratings points, 85
group resources, 52–53
groups: social, 90–91; structural cohesion of, 19

H

H1N1, 7–8
health information, 94–95
health promotion: anti-drug campaigns, 43, 83–84, 84–85, 86–87; anti-smoking campaigns, 26–27, 58–59, 70–71, 79, 86; anti-tobacco advertisements, 26–27; HIV prevention, 34, 59, 70; HIV testing, 59, 68–69; HPV vaccination, 70; Refer a Friend program (Minnesota Department of Health), 27, 33–34, 56–57; via social networks, 11
Higgs Boson ("God particle"), 2–3
high-arousal emotions, 71
Hispanic cultures, 60
HIV prevention, 34, 59, 70
HIV testing campaigns, 68–69
Hong Kong, 61
HPV vaccination, 70
humanity, 20
Hurricane Katrina, 7, 8
Hurricane Sandy, 31, 47, 63

I

i-Neighbors, 101
incentives, financial, 27, 74–75
India, 61
individual differences: that affect information sharing, 31–45; limits of, 44–45
influentials, 48
Influentials Hypothesis, 48
information access: differences in, 7; equal, 94; to health information, 94–95, 102
information age, 3
information diffusion, 12–13
information dissemination, 93–94
information engagement, 35–36
information hubs, 32–33
information sharing: among colleagues, 11; catalogue of behaviors, 17–29, 21*f*; community-level factors that affect, 47–62; community ties and, 54–56; consequences of, 77–91; content-level factors, 63–75; as currency for relationships, 55; differences in, 13–15; diffusion of memes, 68; disparities in, 5–6, 12–13, 13–15, 32, 93–96, 103–106; dissemination of information, 93–94; emotion in, 71–72; energy information sharing, 39; engagement with engagement, 91; equal access to, 94; examples, 2–3; between groups, 8; individual-level factors that affect, 31–45, 67; inequality in, 7–15; initial ideas about, 64–65; many-to-many, 3; message-level differences, 75; multilevel model, 53; between networks, 18; one-to-many, 3; online discussions, 19–20; peer-to-peer, 97–98; perceived understanding and, 39; stories read and e-mailed the most, 64–65, 65*t*, 66*t*; where people are, 98–99; word-of-mouth advertising, 10–11; word-of-mouth epidemics, 11
information utility, 35–36
innovation: adoption of, 50, 77–78, 78–79; medical, 50
inoculation, 88–89
Internet access, 102
interpersonal interactions, 10–11. *see also* social interactions
interpersonal ties, 20

K

Kenya, 59
Kincaid, Judy, 97–98
knowledge gain, 79–81, 89
knowledge gaps, 8–9, 32

L

late adopters, 32
Latinos (or Latinas), 38
leadership, opinion, 32, 40
LED (light-emitting diode) light bulbs, 77–78, 82, 88–89
liking posts, 21, 25
loveLife, 68

M

Madonna, 26
mammography programs, 27, 33–34, 56–57
marketing: credit card, 88–89; designated market areas, 38; interpersonal interactions as tools for, 10–11; science, 98–99; viral, 10–11; word-of-mouth, 10–11, 61
mash ups, 26
mass media campaigns, 82, 85, 86
mass media news coverage, 66
Massachusetts, 26–27
mathematics, 44
McCroskey, James, 40
media campaigns, 82, 85, 86
medical innovation, 50
meme machines, 67–68
memes, 12, 67–68
memory, 81–82, 83–84, 84*f*
messages: as confidence boosters, 72–74; differences in, 75; exposure of, 21*f*; factors related to, 63
Mexico, 61
Minnesota Department of Health, 27, 33–34, 56–57
moderation, 85
Mondale, Walter, 12
motivation, 35–36

N

National Center for Charitable Statistics, 57
National Science Foundation (NSF), 73
the Netherlands, 61, 79
network structure, 9–10, 50–51
networks, 17
The New York Times, 71

New Zealand, 59
news: mass media coverage of, 66; social
    network interactions about, 2–3; stories
    most likely to be forwarded, 67; stories
    read and e-mailed the most, 64–65, 65t,
    66t; stories that boost confidence, 73
News & Observer (Raleigh, North Carolina),
    64, 65, 66t
Next Stop Design project, 55
North Carolina, 14–15
Norway, 70

O
obesity, 89–90
Oklahoma grassfires (2009), 24
online chat, 24–25
online discussion boards, 99–100
online discussion forums, 99–100, 100–101
online discussions, 19–20, 99–100
online support groups, 100
opinion leaders, 32, 40
oral communication, 41. *see also*
    conversation; talk
overt endorsement, 21f, 25–26

P
Page, Larry, 98–99
Patient Protection and Affordable Care Act
    (Affordable Care Act), 1, 2, 64–65
PatientsLikeMe.com, 99, 101
peer referral / referral: examples, 27, 56–57;
    incentives for, 27, 74–75; as information-
    sharing behavior, 21f, 27; innovation
    adoption due to, 78–79; word-of-mouth
    referrals, 61
peer-to-peer communication, 105–106
perceived effectiveness, 61
perceived topical relevance, 36
perceived understanding, 37–39
permissiveness, conversational, 58
personal influence, 47–48
Personal Influence (Katz and Lazarsfeld), 12
personality, 39–40
personality strength, 40
Pete Street, 97–98
Pinterest, 17
Poland, 61
power law distribution, 19
preferential attachment, 13
prescription drugs: promoting, 59, 61–62
procommunity action, 56

protest & denigration, 21f
provocative content, 70
PSY, 12
public health, 14–15
public health campaigns: anti-drug,
    83–84, 86–87; anti-smoking, 70–71, 79;
    examples, 26–27; for HIV testing, 68–69;
    public service announcements, 43, 86–87;
    Refer a Friend program (Minnesota
    Department of Health), 27, 33–34, 56–57;
    word-of-mouth techniques for, 11
public service announcements, 43, 86–87

Q
QuitNet, 101

R
racial background, 38, 102
radio soap operas, 11, 34
realism, 93–108
Red River flooding (spring 2009), 24
Refer a Friend program (Minnesota
    Department of Health), 27, 33–34, 56–57
referrals: examples, 27, 56–57; incentives
    for, 27, 74–75; as information-sharing
    behavior, 21f, 27; innovation adoption
    due to, 78–79; word-of-mouth, 61
relationships: information sharing as
    currency for, 55; past relationship history,
    57–59
relevance, topical, perceived, 36
residential stability, 56–57
resources, 52–53
reticence, 40–41
rhetorical ellipsis, 68–69
rhetorical structure, 68–70
Rhode Island, 14–15
rumor, 71–72
Russia, 61

S
Scandinavian cultures, 60
science: marketing, 98–99; perceived
    understanding of, 37; prevalent
    understandings of, 82–83; talk about,
    39, 44
science education, informal, 98
scientists, 82–83
The Selfish Gene (Dawkins), 12
sensation seeking, 41–44
The Sex Pistols, 26

sharing of information. *see* information sharing
shyness, 40–41
smoking cessation: advertisements for, 26–27, 58–59, 70–71, 86; mass media campaigns, 79; QuitNet, 101
social bonding, 52, 55–56
social capital, 51–53
social clustering, 18–19
social cohesion, 51–53
social groups, 90–91
social interactions: consequences of, 7–8, 89–91; differences in, 8; everyday occurrences, 10–11, 22; examples, 2–3, 7–8; innovation adoption due to, 78–79; manners of, 20; as marketing tool, 10–11
social network sites, 102
social networks, 17–21; availability of, 47–48; building, 99–103; characteristics of, 49–51; connectivity of, 91; definition of, 17; density of, 49–50; importance of, 7–8; information sharing between, 18; linkages between, 18–19; structure of, 9–10, 19, 50–51; talk in, 83–84, 84*f*; unevenness of, 91; as vectors for spread of inoculation, 88–89
social norms, 85–88, 89
social presence, 27–28
social stratification, 35–36
socioeconomic status, 32, 33–34, 102
SolarCity, 27
South Africa, 68–69
strong ties, 20
structural cohesion, 19
support groups, online, 100

T
talk: boosting confidence in, 72–74; as information-sharing behavior, 21*f*, 22–23; online chat, 24–25; online discussions, 19–20, 99–100, 100–101; perceived understanding and, 38–39; planned, 23; preparation for, 80–81; about science or technology, 39, 44; in social networks, 83–84, 84*f*. *see also* conversation
Tanzania, 11, 34
Tarde, Gabriel, 12

technology: adoption of, 50, 77–78, 78–79; communication technologies, 6, 102; connective, 102, 103; talk about, 39, 44
television news: perceived topical relevance in, 36; perceived understanding of, 38
text messages, 56
Thailand, 61
Thanksgiving conversations, 37, 80
tobacco cessation: anti-smoking advertisements, 58–59, 86; anti-tobacco efforts, 26–27, 86
Tobit regression, 57
topics: of e-mailed stories, 64–65, 65*t*, 66*t*; perceived relevance of, 36; of stories read and e-mailed, 65, 66*t*; trending, 31, 63
transportation safety, 34, 35
truncated premise, 68–69
Twitter, 7–8, 24, 31, 63, 103
two-step flow, 80–81

U
understanding: contextual, 62; perceived, 37–39
United States, 61
University of Minnesota, 34
US Department of Health and Human Services (HHS), 25
Usenet conversations, 20
user-focused applications, 103

V
variable interaction, 85
verbal expression. *see* talk
ViaCord, 27
viral communication, 10–11
viral marketing, 10–11
volunteerism, 54

W
Washington Post, 64–65, 65*t*
weak ties, 18–19, 20, 52
WebMD, 99
Wendy's, 12
"Where's the beef?" slogan, 12
whites or Caucasians, 38
word-of-mouth advertising, 10–11
word-of-mouth epidemics, 11
word-of-mouth marketing, 10–11, 61
word-of-mouth referrals, 61